Bach Flower Reflections
from a unique fresh perspective

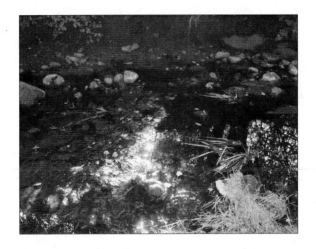

By Sarah Brune, BSc, BFRP
Bach Foundation Registered Practitioner

Note for Librarians:
A cataloguing record for this book is available from Library and Archives Canada at:
www.collectionscanada.ca/amicus/index-e.html
ISBN 978-0-9864748-0-4

Printed at Island Blue Print Company Ltd.
Victoria, British Columbia, Canada

Disclaimer:
All the information presented in this book is for informational purposes only. It is not meant to be a substitute for the advice provided by your own physician or any other medical professional (or veterinarian for animals).

Case history clients have given their full permission to be included in this book, but for confidentiality, their names have been changed.

The remedy descriptions are "reflections" and set out to give a basic understanding of each remedy.

Bach Flower Reflections
from a unique fresh perspective

Contents

Acknowledgements	1
Author's Preface	2
About Dr. Edward Bach	3
Questions and Answers about the Bach Flower Remedies	5
Questions and Answers about Rescue™ Remedy	9
Bach Flower Remedies for Animals	12
Consultations	15
Case Histories	19
Bach Flower Remedy positive and negative indication chart	31
The Thirty-Eight Flower Remedies – some "reflections"	35
Life's Reflections	61
Bibliography	69
Further information	70
About the Author	71
Index	72

Dedication

This book is dedicated to my family,
Mum, Dad, Jane, Karl, Josh, Josie,

and all those who are interested in the Bach Flower Remedies.

Acknowledgements

It was not until I had finished writing the manuscript for this book, that I realized how much help I would need to get it off the ground. Many thanks go to everyone who has helped along the way, giving suggestions, encouragement, and support.
In particular to:

My family:

Karl – you now know which remedies I need!

Josie – as always you have taken an interest in the Bach Flowers, and your illustrations of the flowers are beautiful.

Josh – sorry to disappoint you, but there is no death, or destruction in this book!

Dad – Thank you for taking the time to look through the manuscript, and for all your suggestions.

And friends:

Carol – for going over the manuscript.

Linda – for bringing the book to life with your graphic genius.

Diane – for your continued help and encouragement.

Linda, Ted, Jessie and Maureen (Movers and Shakers) – thanks for being there along the way.

Author's Preface

The idea for writing this book came to me in the fall of 2007, after a particular teaching course that I wanted to attend was unexpectedly cancelled. After it became apparent that no other teaching courses were on the horizon, I decided to write a book about the Bach Flower Remedies instead and the information would be out there for all who wanted it.

I began writing the book in September 2008, working on it in stops and starts. Life got in the way with distractions, and then I started to put hurdles up in front of myself. On October 1, 2009, after taking various remedies and other holistic help, I saw the light at the end of the tunnel for my book. I simply decided to write and it would happen, and that it would be ready to take to England for Christmas.

From writing this book I have learned a lot about the remedies and about myself. I am continuing on my Bach Flower journey and self-healing. I hope that the people's lives that I have touched and guided with the Bach Flowers are a bit better because of it.

The intent of this book is to be a reference guide giving practical advice on all aspects of the Bach Flower Remedies,* for their everyday use for people and pets alike. Dr. Bach created a simple system of self-healing, and that is what I hope to get across, from a unique fresh "reflective" perspective.

*More information is available from the Bach Centre - www.bachcentre.com

About Dr. Edward Bach

"They cure, not by attacking the disease, but by flooding our bodies with the beautiful vibrations of our Higher Nature, in the presence of which, disease melts away as snow in the sunshine. There is no true healing unless there is a change in outlook, peace of mind and inner happiness." – Dr. Edward Bach 1934. Howard, J. and Ramsell, J. *The Original Writings of Edward Bach.*

Dr. Edward Bach was born on September 24, 1886 in Moseley England. From 1906-1912 he studied medicine at the University College Hospital in London and trained as a doctor. By 1922 Dr. Bach worked in a general practice out of consulting rooms in Harley Street, having also studied bacteriology, immunology, and homeopathy during his career.

Over time, he realized that people reacted differently to illnesses, so he wanted to treat the person as a whole rather than what they were suffering from. Dr. Bach became dissatisfied with orthodox medicine and was convinced there must be a system of healing based purely in nature. So in 1930 he gave up his lucrative Harley Street Practice and left London, determined to devote his time to a new system that surely could be found in nature.

Relying on intuition and his natural gifts as a healer to guide him, he spent many years searching for and developing his system from non-poisonous plants and flowers. Gradually, one by one, these were found to assist with a particular emotion or mental state.

For several years he spent the summers searching for and preparing the remedies, and winters helping patients. In 1934, Dr. Bach moved to Sotwell in Oxfordshire, where he lived in a small house called Mount Vernon. There he created a centre for his work, discovering the remaining remedies to complete the series in the garden and surrounding countryside.

After the discovery of the 38 remedies in 1936, Dr. Bach announced his work was complete. On his 50th birthday, September 24th, 1936, he published his final works and gave his

3

first public lecture, entitled 'Healing by Herbs,' at the Masonic Lodge in Wallingford.

He died on November 27 of that year, knowing that he had completed his work by devising a simple self-help form of healing covering all aspects of human nature's moods. His system is now available and used in most parts of the world.

Mount Vernon is now the **Bach Centre** and his trustees still collect and prepare the plants for the Mother Tinctures in the same simple way as Dr. Bach intended.

The Bach system is made up of 38 healing plants addressing the different states of mind. The remedies help the physical body to gain strength and assist the mind to become calm, widen its outlook, and strive towards perfection, thus bringing peace and harmony to the whole personality.

Dr. Bach's philosophy:

- A healthy mind is the key to recovery, and the remedies work by gently restoring balance to negative emotions
- The key is to cure the personality, because different personality types react to illness and cope with it in different ways. The remedies deal with the personalities i.e. treating the patient and not the disease
- Everyone has a purpose in life, but often gets lost on the way. The remedies help us to become our true selves and to rediscover our true purpose in life. Health and true healing would soon follow
- Dr. Bach intended his system to be a simple self-help measure available to people from all walks of life

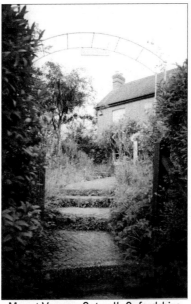
Mount Vernon, Sotwell, Oxfordshire

Questions and Answers about the Bach Flower Remedies

How are the remedies made?

The flowers of the plants, trees, and bushes used are mainly found in the garden at the Bach Centre and in the surrounding countryside. Many of the locations are the ones that Dr. Bach himself used.

The Sun Method is used for the more delicate flowers that bloom in the height of the summer. The flowers are carefully picked and then placed in a glass bowl of spring water. They are left floating on top of the water in the direct sunlight for three hours.

For the woodier, hardier plants and flowers that bloom later in the year when the sun is not so strong, the Boiling Method is used. The plants and flowers are placed in a saucepan and boiled for half an hour, and then taken outside to cool.

The filtered prepared water from both methods is then mixed

50/50 with full strength 40% brandy (used as a preservative), and this mix is known as the mother tincture. Two drops of the mother tincture are further diluted at the ratio of two drops to 30 ml. of brandy, the finished product being the stock bottles.

Due to the growing demand for the remedies, after the mother tincture is made at the Bach Centre, Nelsons now carry out the bottling and distribution. At Nelsons the stock bottles are sealed for quality and safety and dispatched to stores around the world.

How do the remedies work?

The Bach Flower Remedies work by subtly restoring balance to negative emotions, such as stress, depression, and fear. Two drops of the appropriate remedy can assist with restoring equilibrium.

How do I know which ones to take?

In Dr. Bach's words: *"Take no notice of the disease, think only of the outlook on life of the one in distress."* Since Dr. Bach intended his remedies to be a simple system of self-healing, it was his hope that *"There should be no difficulty either for oneself or another, to find that state or a mixture of states which are present, and so be able to give the required remedies to effect a cure."* (Dr. Edward Bach, *The Twelve Healers and Other Remedies*)

What is the dosage?

For immediate use for passing moods, simply take two drops of the remedy of your choice or four drops of Rescue™ Remedy from a stock bottle either by mouth or in a glass of water. This can be sipped at intervals until symptoms improve.

For longer-term use, up to seven remedies (two drops of each selected remedy and four drops of Rescue™ Remedy) of your choice can be added to a 30 ml. dropper bottle, topped up with mineral water. Four drops of this solution can be taken as often as needed, but at least four times a day, especially first thing in the morning and last thing at night.

How are the remedies administered?

The drops can be taken directly into the mouth, or added to the beverage of your choice. They are not affected by smells, flavours, or heat. Alternatively, add ten to twelve drops to your bath water or four drops to a water mister. Four drops can be taken from the treatment bottle and added to a drink container for use throughout the day.

How long do I take them for?

The remedies can be taken as often as needed, and there is no chance of overdosing. If they are not needed they will not work. Taken regularly, the remedies in the treatment bottle should last for approximately three weeks. Either keep in a fridge or add some brandy as a preservative. When the bottle is empty, it is a good time to review the mix of remedies. You can stop taking the remedies when you no longer feel the need for them.

Are the remedies safe for every family member to use?

Yes, they are safe for the whole family – babies, children, nursing mothers, and the elderly. If you have any concerns always seek the advice of a health professional. If the inactive ingredient of brandy is a problem, simply dilute, boil, use it externally, or refrain from use.

Are the remedies safe for pets?

Yes, simply add to their water, food, or treat, or place behind the ears, on the paws or directly into the mouth (dilute due to alcohol content). My dogs lick it off my hand. If you are concerned about your pet's health, always consult a veterinarian, as the remedies are not meant to replace medical attention.

How do I reduce the alcohol intake of the remedies?

Since the stock remedies are preserved in alcohol and there is a trace of alcohol (twenty-seven per cent grape alcohol solution) in each dosage, some suggestions are:

- Dilute the drops in juice or water, or add to a water mister, or add ten to twelve drops to a bath
- Apply them externally on the temples, wrists, or behind the ears
- Put the remedies in a pot of water and boil until the alcohol content is evaporated
- If it is still an issue, refrain from use

Are there any side effects?

No. There are no known adverse reactions from using the remedies. The remedies are non-addictive and there are no known side effects. If a particular remedy is not needed it will not take effect.

However, they may allow suppressed symptoms to surface. This is an important part of the healing process, and is only temporary. The remedies are not used to suppress negative attitudes, but do transform them into positive ones, stimulating self-healing. If you have any concerns always seek the advice of a health professional.

Can the remedies be taken in conjunction with medical or other treatments?

Yes. They will not conflict, influence, or affect any other medication or treatments. The remedies act on the emotional level; not the physical. Please note they are not intended to be a substitute for medical treatment, and always consult your medical practitioner if you are in any doubt.

How long can I keep my stock bottles for?

The actual stock remedies essentially keep forever. The brandy it is preserved in has a shelf life of five years, hence the expiry date on the label.

Questions and Answers about Rescue™ Remedy

In the 1930 Dr. Bach combined five specific remedies from the 38 for a composite that he called "Rescue™ Remedy." Today it is probably the most used and well-known Bach Flower product.

What is Rescue™ Remedy?

Rescue™ Remedy is a mix of five different Bach Flower Remedies, which together help deal with any stressful or emergency situation. The purpose being to treat the pre- and post-emotional effect that is experienced through shock, fear, panic, stress, etc.

What is in Rescue™ Remedy?

Cherry Plum - is for hysteria or loss of self-control - *If you have temper tantrums, hysteria, hyperactivity, sudden outrages, are abnormally abusive, or feel as if you are about to explode, have PMS, or feel that you are on the verge of a breakdown, or fearful of releasing emotions etc.* - It helps with calmness and composure.

Clematis - is for faintness/dreaminess - *Dreamy, unable to concentrate, dizziness, absentmindedness, inattentiveness, lethargy, etc.* - It assists with focus.

Impatiens - is for undue agitation - *When you are irritated by other people's slowness, or are always in a hurry, and want things to happen or to be done right now, if you are restless, and talk and think quickly, or are hyperactive, short-tempered etc.* - It assists with patience.

Rock Rose - is for terror and or panic - *Thunderstorms, certain insects and animals, going to the dentist, flying, having an operation, exams, public speaking, interviews, the dark, night terrors, heights, claustrophobia, anxiety attacks, separation anxiety etc.* - It helps create peace and fearlessness.

Star of Bethlehem - is for shock and trauma (timeless) - *Receiving bad news, after being stung by an insect, emergency situation such as a car accident, loss of a job, death of a loved one, etc.* - Assists with comfort and consolation.

Are there any other ingredients?

Yes. The remedies are preserved in the inactive ingredient, a twenty-seven per cent grape alcohol solution.

What forms does it come in?

Rescue™ Remedy is available in a dropper, in a convenient spray, or in a soft, non-greasy cream that contains the added benefits of Crab Apple that can help heal rashes, minor cuts and bruises.

When do I use Rescue™ Remedy?

It is best to use it in an emergency or in stressful situations. If you tend to use it all the time or frequently you may want to look if any of the other 38 remedies would suit you better.

How do I administer it?

Rescue™ Remedy can be taken neat from the bottle, four drops or two sprays at a time either directly under the tongue, or on pulse points. Otherwise, put four drops or two sprays in a glass of water and take frequent sips until the emotions have calmed. If for some reason the recipient is unable to swallow, simply use four drops to moisten the lips, or behind the ears or on the inside of the wrists.

How long before it works?

It can work instantly. However, if you have an interview coming up, or some sort of situation you are not looking forward to, you can start using it the day before.

Can it be used alongside the other 38 remedies?

Yes. All 38 of the remedies including the five remedies used in Rescue™ Remedy, can be taken equally effectively separately as required.

Is it safe for every family member to use?

Yes, it is safe for the whole family – babies, children, nursing mothers, and the elderly. If you have any concerns always seek the advice of a health professional. If the inactive alcohol ingredient is a problem, simply dilute, boil or use it externally. Alternatively use Rescue Cream.

Is it safe for pets?

Yes, simply add to their water, food, or treat, or place behind their ears, on their paws, or directly into the mouth. It is preserved in alcohol, but can be diluted. If you are concerned about your pet's health, always consult a veterinarian, as it is not meant to replace medical attention.

Are there any side effects?

There are no known side effects. It is safe, gentle and non-habit forming. Rescue™ Remedy does not interfere with other medications. Please speak with a health professional if you have any concerns.

Is it intended to replace medical attention?

Absolutely not. Rescue™ Remedy is not intended to replace medical attention or care. It does, however, keep everyone calm when waiting for and/or receiving medical attention.

Is it safe to take if I am on any other form of medication?

Yes, it is safe and compatible. If you have any concerns always speak to your health professional.

"When my son was a little nervous about the ceremony for entering into Beavers I offered him a "squirt" of the Rescue Remedy. He said he felt better and showed no signs of apprehension. Later that evening when I was tucking him in he said "I'm afraid of the dark ... can I have some of that Rescue Remedy".... I left the bottle on his night stand and all was peaceful." **Judy**

"I found the Rescue Remedy to be helpful prior to exam writing and public speaking. On the same day I wrote an exam and gave a presentation, a little Rescue Remedy beforehand seemed to calm my nerves and allow me to focus on what I had to do." **Ross**

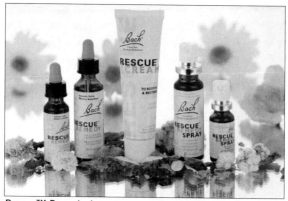

Rescue™ Remedy drops, cream, and spray. Photo by Sarah Kerr

Bach Flowers for Animals

Animals have emotions too, and are subject to the same stresses and emotional challenges that can affect humans. The Bach Flower Remedies offer a gentle means of relieving negative attitudes, providing a harmless, non-habit forming system of healing. Animals often react quickly and positively to the remedies, which are suitable for animals of all ages and sizes.

The Bach Flower Remedies can help animals cope with everyday stressful situations or certain behaviours. For example:

- Break bad habits with Chestnut Bud
- Remove territoriality issues with Vine
- Reduce jealousy with Holly
- Eliminate fear and stress with Mimulus
- Relieve the effects of change with Walnut
- Calm overactive or tense behaviour with Vervain

"I am just writing to you to you to let you know what I have experienced with using Bach Flowers for our dogs. Our dog has been pretty excitable in the past and I have been using one of your remedy mixtures and we have noticed at how much calmer he has become. He loves taking the mixture right out of the palm of my hand. As soon as he sees the bottle he comes over to me wagging his tail. He has had to

have surgery recently and the mixture that you have given us for him for that has helped him with the healing. He is much easier to handle and more controllable yet none of these have changed his personality. One of our dogs used to suffer from separation anxiety and after giving her some Bach Flowers we have not noticed her acting the way she used to at all anymore." **Cheryl from Comox**

Rescue™ Remedy is a mix of five different Bach Flower Remedies that together deal with a variety of stressful or emergency situations. It can assist animals with remaining calm and in control. For example:

- Visits to the vet
- Adapting to new surroundings
- Fear of loud noises
- Excessive barking or hissing
- Separation anxiety
- Shock, trauma or mistreatment
- Obsessive cleansing
- Any emergency situation

"The product (Rescue Remedy) worked very well in helping to move our cat with more ease. She moved to another city with my daughter, and it was a very stressful and traumatic experience for the cat. My daughter said the drops really, really helped because of the calming, relaxing affect they had on the cat during the car ride, and for the next week or so, until the cat got accustomed to the new surroundings." **Ida R**

Selection

Selecting remedies for animals can be a challenge. Look for changes in their behaviour that can be due to changes of daily routines, new situations, or events – new job, new family member or pet, a move, injury, or even an operation. Try to put yourself in their position and empathize with how your pet feels. For a more detailed analysis of the situation a consultation by a Bach Foundation Registered Practitioner is an option. If in doubt about the health of your pet seek the advice of a veterinarian.

Dosage

The dosage is two drops from each selected remedy, or four drops of Rescue™ Remedy. Always dilute before use, since it is preserved in brandy. For any medical concerns always seek the advice from a veterinarian.

For longer-term use a treatment bottle can be made up. Add two drops of each individual remedy and four of Rescue™ Remedy (up to seven max) to a 30 ml. bottle of spring water. A dose is four drops from this bottle, and you should give at least four doses a day. Use until symptoms improve. There are many ways to give the remedies to animals, so pick the one that works for you.

- Drip the remedies onto pads, paws, nose, or ears so they will be absorbed through the skin or licked off
- You can put the remedies into food, onto pet treats, or in their water
- If pets share water, the remedies won't have any effects on the other pets if they don't need them
- For larger animals adjust the dosage according to their size
- There is no worry of overdosing

Please note: The remedies will not change the inherent temperament of a particular breed or animal, but will help bring it into balance. The remedies do not treat any medical conditions directly. If you are in any doubt about the health of your pet, seek the advice of a veterinarian.

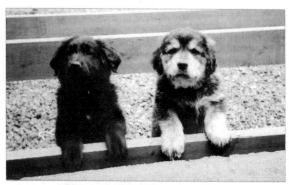

Alice and Harry Brune as puppies

Consultations

What are the purposes and benefits of a consultation?

The purpose of a consultation with a trained Bach Flower practitioner is to have a one-on-one, preferably face-to-face, meeting to discuss what is going on in the client's world, in order to determine which remedies are required at that time. The role of the practitioner is to be their guide, listen to what they have to say, and then make suggestions as to which remedies can assist.

The client is in no way obligated to take those particular remedies, and has an opportunity to go through a chart or book to see what jumps out at them. The practitioner will explain the implications of each remedy and how it fits in with their particular situation.

Remedies can also be self-selected by the client as they are a simple system of self-healing, which is what Dr. Bach intended. However, sometimes it is beneficial to discuss with someone else what their current situation is so they can "get it off their chest" in a confidential, quiet and tranquil setting. This discussion can begin the healing process.

This is summed up in an email I received from a client's mother, after I did a consultation over the phone and then sent out the remedies to them.

"The remedies arrived in the middle of last week, but they started working before then! Gillian has been so taken by the whole process that there has been a change in her already. I think it is to do with the acknowledgement that certain emotional issues exist for her and the attention and sense of being special that treating them has brought for her." **Alice K**

Once a list of remedy choices is compiled, each remedy's positive potential and how it related to the clients particular situation are discussed. Sometimes as many as twenty remedies have come up, but by going through them and ruling out ones that can be left for now, six or seven remedies are then selected.

Two drops of each chosen remedy are put into a 30 ml. bottle and topped up with spring water. Four drops are then to be taken four times a day until the bottle is finished, in approximately three weeks. The remedies can be dropped directly into the mouth, added to any beverage, or food, and even added to bath water. No taste or smell can affect them.

If the client wishes to come back for a follow-up consultation, the previous personal blend of remedies is discussed to see if there is any change in their situation, and if any particular remedies are to be repeated. On these subsequent visits fewer remedies seem to be discussed, often; twelve as opposed to twenty or more.

After seeing clients over a year or so, it is encouraging to see the results; how the emotional layers have shed (like the layers of an onion) and their situation has improved. Someone may come to me because of a particular unpleasant event that has taken place or maybe they are just at their wits' end. With the assistance of the remedies, over time, the conversation is more around their day-to-day life. A bit of fine-tuning with additional remedies is done to make their life or situation easier.

A client may come because of one particular reason, and as the conversation goes on more and more things seem to crop up. I am amazed at how much emotional baggage people are dealing with. Very often they have been suffering for years.

The practitioner is the guide knowing the indications of the remedies, and applying them to a specific situation. If a client cannot sleep, there is no one remedy**, nor is there for stress. Each client is unique. Sleeplessness or stress may be caused by many factors, some stemming back years and years. The remedies are by no means a quick fix, and work subtly; some clients explain things as "lightning bolts out of the blue." There may be small changes at first that lead onto bigger things like deciding what you really want to do. Suddenly, without realizing it, you are where you really want to be, doing what you love. For others, their whole life has had a turnaround for the better***.

A good example of this is my friend Sue, whom I met traveling in the late 1980s.

May 2003 – Testimonial – *"After taking the remedies I found that I was having "bolts out of the blue," sudden decisive thoughts coming into my head from nowhere. I would think, "Why didn't I think of that before?" Things seemed simpler, almost as though my mind was untangling the knots of thoughts that were built up. I have only been taking the remedies for two days so I feel that gradually the answers that I'm seeking will become clearer, as the "knots" untangle. I can already feel myself being more confident in my ability to make decisions and to know what I need instead of relying on everybody else to tell me what they want me to do!"* **Sue**

May 2003 – Her entry in my visitor's book
"It has been ten years since my last entry in this book, and I'm back again – I keep wafting through. Unfortunately, my life is no more settled and I am still a "Spinster of the Parish." I have spent the last month with an old boyfriend, and am going back up there tomorrow for six weeks. It's make it or break it time! I'm not sure which way it will go. I'll either live happily ever after or head back to the UK in mid-June to look for a job in remotest Scotland where I can gaze out to sea, make furniture out of driftwood, and learn to play the bagpipes. Who knows? Sarah has been loading me up with Bach Flower Remedies, desperately trying to bring some meaning and direction into my poor, sad, directionless life. I live in hope that I may suddenly have a "lightning bolt" moment and know where I am going." **Sue**

A few months later, my family and I went over to England for a visit, and hoped to be able to meet up with Sue. When we got to the UK she called to say she could not see me because she was going back to Fair Isle, Scotland (Britain's most remote inhabited island), to work at the Bird Observatory because they were short staffed.

The next time I heard from Sue, she said she had met someone and was engaged. It was then that I remembered her entry in our visitor's book. I called Sue to tell her about it, and what a coincidence it was. Some time later I called her mother to talk about her engagement and the entry in my visitor's book. Her mother said if she had known there was such a simple solution, she would have given her some remedies years ago. 2009 - Sue is still engaged, living in a croft, and cooking lunches for the school children in Fair Isle.

It is just a matter of going on your journey of self-healing to discover the aspects of your life that you can do without, and make your life better for yourself. Remove the barriers, such as fear, lack of confidence, worry, guilt, and influence from others that stop you from getting on in the world. Once you break through them you will be able to reach your true potential, whether it is life on a remote Scottish Island or turning a passion into a successful career – it is your life. You choose. No strings attached!

In addition, the remedies can be used for passing moods or to get you through a particular day. They can help you to feel more relaxed, more fulfilled, and ultimately, better prepared for whatever life may throw your way.

"We are all healers, and with love and sympathy in our natures we are also able to help anyone who really desires health." (Howard, J. and Ramsell, J. *The Original Writings of Edward Bach*)

** *"I began working with Sarah in November 2004 because of insomnia and the anxiety accompanied by sleeplessness. I used three different combinations of Bach Remedies over three months (Vervain, Walnut, Chestnut Bud, and Mimulus). Initially the remedies did not seem to affect me much. However, in January 2005, my insomnia lifted – I began to sleep more regularly, and for longer hours, which affected my working life. I now feel more grounded with regard to my work, which can, at times, feel overwhelming. My overall mood is more positive and, in general, I feel a lightness and sense of well-being that has been lacking in the past four to five months. Thank you, Sarah and thank you, Dr. Bach."* **Judy**

*** *"When I began the Bach Remedies I was feeling completely depressed, useless, and tired. I was always making excuses to do* *nothing and for why I did nothing. But after only a few days of taking my first remedy family and friends already noticed a change in me and that change only progressed. Now I feel like I've had a 360 degrees change and I'm feeling better now than I ever have. Not only that, but the people in my family seem to have changed from it as well."* **Caroline**

Case Histories

Margaret's case history

Margaret – dog trainer in her mid-forties, common law partner, and two grown-up girls.

In mid-October, 2008, Margaret was going through a traumatic time, due to a distressing incident. I suggested adding some remedies to her drinking water, including **Walnut** for protection.

A few weeks later, Margaret started another treatment of remedies to help her continue to deal with a distressing saga. Due to the fact that the emotional trauma continued, I suggested to Margaret that some consultations might be an option. She signed up as a case-study client.

December 4, 2008

Margaret thought she was having a meltdown. She was feeling depressed and was having trouble getting out of bed. She felt exhausted. For several months, she had been going through a bad patch dealing with a very unpleasant situation, particularly fueled by one person.

There was a lot of grief and depression coming out of nowhere. The last time Margaret had felt like this was when her father died two years ago, and then she slept for long periods of time. Everything seemed normal. Then a black cloud of depression descended upon her. She felt sapped from exhaustion and lack of enthusiasm. The thought of an upcoming meeting made her feel terrified about losing her temper, and about being humiliated. Despite this fear, Margaret thought it necessary to go to the meeting.

Twelve remedies were discussed. The remedies chosen to assist with her depression were **Sweet Chestnut** because she felt miserable and bleak with despair, and Olive to give her sufficient energy to get through her days. For the upcoming meeting – **Walnut** to protect her from outside influences, **Cherry Plum** so she would remain calm and not lose control, **Rock Rose** to relieve the terror of being humiliated, and **Larch** for confidence.

January 30, 2009

When I next met with Margaret a month later, she was suffering from panic attacks, and the feelings of being overwhelmed. Her partner had been away for several weeks, which had not helped. In general, she was feeling flustered and short tempered.

Larch, Olive, and **Sweet Chestnut** were repeated. **Hornbeam** was added to assist with procrastination and **Elm** for the feelings of being overwhelmed.

March 24, 2009

At our next meeting a few months later, Margaret was feeling stressed and anxious but she was not sure why. The depression and self-pity were still there. Her life was lacking joy. On the business front, Margaret wanted to make some changes. She also felt as though she needed a change.

Larch, Olive, Sweet Chestnut and **Hornbeam** were repeated. **Wild Oat** was given for direction in life and **Willow** to assist with the feelings of self-pity and resentment.

April 21, 2009

A month later Margaret was in a panic about her business, and terrified about her financial situation. All the remedies chosen this time were for being overwrought, in particular **Rock Rose** for terror.

September 30, 2009

Five months later when we next met, things were looking up on the business front and she was no longer overwrought. In general, she was not worrying about things so much and was focusing more on restructuring her business, wanting to focus on dog consultations.

She had some ideas from a business consultant, and was trying to keep to a time schedule, so she could focus on her business more. Margaret was now more organized. As a result, business was picking up.

Margaret felt that she lacked confidence to make cold calls, but once she picked up the phone and got chatting all was fine. Things were taking shape and she felt that there was more direction and clarity in her life. People were coming to see her for their dog consultations, and she was planning to hire a local student for more menial tasks.

There had been a huge turnaround since this time last year, and her attitude had changed considerably. The depression continued, and she was suffering from headaches, which could be linked with her menstrual cycle. Margaret felt as though she had hit "middle-aged woman" status. Since having stopped smoking some time ago, she was in the habit of eating junk food at night, and wanted to be able to break that habit.

Margaret was having problems with getting out of bed, and felt so exhausted by the afternoon that she needed a short nap. "Waking up in the morning is like walking through thick jello and finding it impossible to think." In an ideal world she would like to go to bed at 1:00 a.m. and get up at 10:00 a.m., but instead she had to go to bed at 11:00 p.m. and get up at 7:00 a.m. One reason for broken sleep was sharing the bed with numerous "boarding" dogs.

There was no "down time," and even though Friday was meant to be her day off, it did not seem to happen. When clients asked to drop their dogs off at "all hours," Margaret was unable to say "no" in case she lost their business. Margaret seemed to be busy all the time, and on the rare occasions that her three phones were switched off, she felt guilty. Sometimes there was resentment towards the boarding dogs because they came in the way of any free time. Despite being exhausted she struggled on.

The remedies chosen were to help her "fine tune" her day, so that she would be in control of her day and to make it more bearable. **Centaury, Larch,** and **Mimulus** were chosen to give her the courage and ability to have some time to herself. **Elm** was chosen to help prevent her from being overwhelmed, **Willow** to deal with the resentment, and **Chestnut Bud** to break bad habits. **Oak** was added so she would be able to let herself relax and not struggle on regardless.

Case history summary

All in all, Margaret's life seemed to have changed completely over the past year, and she had endured some troubled unpleasant times, leaving her depressed and overwrought. Over the months, with the depression slowly lifting, Margaret was able to concentrate more on her business making it run more smoothly and efficiently. With the financial and emotional hurdles smoothed out it was now time to "fine tune" and take control of her life, taking time out to relax and have a good night's sleep.

Margaret's testimonial – October 10, 2009

"November, 2008 had some extremely stressful moments in it. Sarah was there for one of them and mixed me up a batch of remedies that I'm pretty sure kept me sane. I remember telling her that it felt like there was a warm and secure blanket that was just draped over my shoulders and helped me centre and relax so that I could continue. Over the past year, Sarah and I have met for consultations and as my life was changing, so were the remedies Sarah put together for me. They say that when the remedy is right, the patient remembers to take it and I always remembered to reach for my remedies. Thanks so much, Sarah, for all your support during this past year." **Margaret N**

Nancy's case history.
Single mother, early 50s, business owner.

December 2007

Nancy came to me in early December, 2007 and explained that she had been feeling overwhelmed for about a year and a half. There had been changes of location and work. She questioned her self-reliance. It had been a difficult time, but tried to stay strong for the sake of her teenage son.

The main issues discussed were sleeping difficulties and the tendency to wake up at 4:30 a.m. She would lie awake for some time and that made it difficult to get up in the morning. Up until four months ago, she had been an early riser.

Right now Nancy was in a quandary of whether to move back East or stay put for the sake of her son. Courage was needed to move forward, to work on her business, and to be financially organized. Currently going through menopause, she felt as though she had visually aged over the last year.

During the consultation eighteen remedies were discussed, and the ones that were chosen were **Wild Oat** for true vocation in life, **Elm** for being overwhelmed as there was so much change, **Walnut** to cope with the change, **Hornbeam** for procrastination, **Scleranthus** for decision-making, and finally **White Chestnut** for the thoughts going around and around. Rescue Remedy was to be taken separately.

January 2008

The second consultation took place a month later and the remedy mix had been taken regularly. Nancy had been experiencing clear dreams at times, and felt as though things were being worked out through the dreams.

Decisions were being made, but the wrong way. After giving her son an electronic device that he wanted for Christmas, she soon regretted it because it was as if a monster had entered the house. Although money was tight she wanted to please her son. She felt awful for falling into that trap.

There was a sense of loss and sorrow, and wanting to be able to take steps, but too much had to be accomplished. Nancy wanted to be the provider and wanted a better place for them both. Generally, she was feeling down and not good enough for anybody.

The sleeping issues had not sorted themselves out. She was still waking up in the early hours, and thoughts kept going around and around. Consequently it was hard to drag herself out of bed, and she was procrastinating.

Nancy was still not certain of what to do. She had been working on a farm and working at her business, and, was anxious about her next step. She never imagined that her depressions could last so long. She doubted her many talents and was still not sure of what direction in life she was seeking. There was also anxiety about doing nothing.

The remedies that were repeated were **Walnut** for change, **Scleranthus** for decision-making, and **Wild Oat** for direction in life. The remaining remedies chosen were **Red Chestnut** for concern for others, **Wild Rose** to put the spark back in life, **White Chestnut** to assist with the thoughts going around and around, and **Willow** for resentment.

April 2008

At our third meeting two months later, she said the dreams were very vivid and when she awoke in the night concerns came rushing in. Nancy had spent time at the Job Shop and was considering her options. Unfortunately she had hurt her heel while working.

She had been having difficulties with her son, and was often more irritated with him than she would have liked. The feelings of inadequacy and of not being a sufficient provider were still there, but she was in the process of selling some property. There was a possibility of visiting a friend back East in May.

The remedies repeated were **Scleranthus** for decision-making, and **Wild Oat** for her life's path. The other remedies chosen were **Mimulus** for worries about her foot, **Gentian** for disappointment, **Agrimony** for hiding her worries behind a cheerful face, and Sweet Chestnut for seeing the light at the end of the tunnel. These remedies were repeated in May. For a short trip in May, **Larch** and **Walnut** were taken.

November 2008

This was the last consultation, and Nancy was experiencing feelings of love and gratitude. Nancy felt a lot better and commented that she was talking a lot. The relationship with her son was better, but she was still a bit irritable and there were some angry interludes. Organization and de-cluttering were well on the way, and she was making steps with her own business.

This time three previous remedies were selected; **Hornbeam** for procrastination, **Elm** for being overwhelmed, and **Walnut** for change. The others being **Vervain** for being over-enthusiastic, **Impatiens** for patience, **Chestnut Bud** to help her not to repeat the same mistakes (cleaning up, etc.), and **Olive** to assist with energy. In addition, a separate bottle of **Heather** was selected to assist with being overly chatty.

Case history summary

Nancy participated in the Level One Bach Flower introductory course (April 2008), and subsequently purchased a Bach Flower Remedy kit, so she can use the remedies whenever the need arises. I am happy to have led her through her Bach Flower journey, and I am pleased that life is easier and more enjoyable for her.

Depression, change, vocation in life, and decision-making seemed to be her main stumbling blocks. Despite the bumps in the road, Nancy found her path in life smoothed by the remedies, and became more at peace within herself.

Nancy's testimonial - April 4, 2009

"More than one year ago, I sought out Sarah Brune, to counsel me and to administer Bach flower essences.

A year before that I had been attracted to her work when I spoke with her at a "healing fair". Sarah's way of being, her soft spoken words, her sense of self assurance around everything that has been offered to the world through Dr. Bach, and the way she managed to keep focused and attentive even amidst a crowd, impressed me favourably.

One year later, after I had tried other things, including a trip to a mental health facility where they suggested anti-depressants, I remembered Sarah, and although I was feeling almost hopeless, I called her.

The first time I was greeted by Sarah in her studio, I felt nurtured. I did have difficulty narrowing my choice of remedies down to seven, as I felt I suffered from most of the conditions of malaise addressed by Dr. Bach. I was skeptical as to whether anything could help me. Although I could remember feeling depressed before, it had never been this severe or this prolonged.

On an average day, I would lie in bed until I had to get up, then I would slowly build a little confidence, so that, by evening, I felt almost myself, at which point I went to bed, slept fitfully, and then start the tedious process over again. I fit right into the Myth of Sisyphus, spending each day rolling a boulder to the top of a mountain only to have it roll back down and necessitate my starting again the following day to push the same heavy boulder up the same daunting slope. I took my remedies and saw Sarah again a month later. Again it was hard to choose; only I was interested to notice that a few of the old ones could be replaced with new ones. I had begun the process of peeling back the layers of the onion.

By the third visit I was aware of a few changes in my life. I had some steady clients for my own business in my new location and had found several new reasons for dwelling where I did. I was still having arguments; only I trusted the remedies to be of help and was able more quickly to recover perspective.

Half a year later I made a decision: to infuse creativity into this new phase of my life, and to drop resentment as I tended to my own priorities. I can now report that a number of things that were weighing me down have shifted, and freedom and autonomy have emerged. I've taken additional training, love my work, and I'm happy with my relations both near and far.

Throughout the process I saw Sarah and adjusted remedies with her help. The last time we had determined a full slate for my bottle, and then I remembered the need for another one, Heather, and Sarah made up a separate bottle with just that, as it helps when a person is feeling overly excited and tending to talk too much, dominating *conversation. And this was now appropriate for me, while months earlier, before I first saw Sarah, I had been afraid to speak!*

I took an introductory training in Bach Flower Essences, which was organized by Sarah. I have now purchased the complete Bach Flower Essences kit so I can self administer and help friends with the remedies." **Nancy**

Anne's case history
Anne, mid-fifties, married with three children. Had been a nurse for the last 35 years.

October 1, 2007
Anne contacted me in late September 2007 after reading an article I wrote about the Bach Flowers, putting a call out for case history clients. Having had a multitude of problems over the last few years and suffering from stress and depression, she wanted to give the Bach Flowers a try. The past year she had taken off work to try to feel better.

Anne's youngest son was heavily into drugs and this was creating an emotional roller coaster of stress. After paying for treatment, he did not follow through with it. In addition his girlfriend was pregnant. Anne and her eldest son did not want him to visit. Her eldest son was married with children whom Anne enjoyed seeing, and her daughter was getting married soon.

The anti-depressants that she had been on for a year were managing to have a calming effect, but she did not like the side effects. She was also concerned about her weight and tended to eat when she was not hungry.

In addition, Anne had been having trouble with an irritable bladder since the age of thirteen. The pills that she had been taking since March seemed to be working, but she had stopped taking them weeks ago. Recently she had been working in the garden, but always felt tired. All in all everything seemed to be piling up.

Sixteen remedies were discussed at length, and the ones chosen were **Wild Oat** for purpose in life, **Crab Apple** for feeling better about herself, **Beech** for intolerance, **Chestnut Bud** for breaking bad habits, **Holly** for anger, **Olive** for energy to get her through the day, and **Walnut** for protection against outside influences.

October 25, 2007

On her second visit later that month, Anne reported that she still felt critical of others, and continued to eat all the time. On the plus side she was not so worried about her weight, was feeling more positive and less tired. Anne was getting over the flu. Her husband had mentioned that she had been snoring, and she was still experiencing bladder problems.

The remedies repeated were **Beech, Chestnut Bud, Holly, Olive**, and **Walnut**. The two new ones chosen were **Impatiens** for patience, and **Wild Rose** for some spark in her life.

November 1, 2007

Anne self-selected the next batch of remedies and selected two bottles. She chose **Beech** for intolerance, **Chicory** for over-protection, **Holly** for anger, **Impatiens** for patience, **Pine** for guilt, and **Walnut** for change.

When she talked to me a few months later, she commented that she had been having dreams about people she knew going further and further into her past. They were good dreams.

June 2008

I checked in with Anne in June 2008. She was feeling calmer and did not recall having any more dreams.

October 15, 2008

There had been a long gap since we last got together, and so we discussed how the last set of remedies were helping. Anne felt as though she was more tolerant, more patient, generally feeling better, and she had stopped taking sleeping pills. Her bladder seemed worse and was still a problem, and the pills she was taking did not seem to be helping. She thought that the trauma she had experienced in her teenage years might have been a factor because that is when she started to have bladder problems. As far as her son was concerned Anne was coping better and feeling more peaceful about him being in jail. She felt less guilty about things and was beginning to let go.

The **Walnut** seemed to be helping with protecting her from outside influences and she did not let things bother her. She was not taking more things on. She had been off anti-depressants for three months, and felt more alive and generally not too bad as she could "feel again." On the whole she was managing a lot better, and things seemed to have changed for the better. For the past couple of weeks she had been dreaming about people she knew, but the dreams were not unpleasant.

The remedies repeated were **Chestnut Bud** to break bad habits, **Beech** for intolerance, and **Walnut** for protection from change. New remedies this time were **Vine** to assist with bossiness, and **Star of Bethlehem** for shock and trauma.

January 9, 2009

When I next met with Anne in January she had been taking new anti-depressants but had stopped taking them three months ago because she did not like them. In general, she was feeling more peaceful, but her bladder was not any better. Her son was in jail again and this was making her depressed. When he called Anne did not answer the phone, and she was wondering how she would get through this. She was thinking of going back on anti-depressants.

That week she had started to do voluntary work and had an upsetting incident at work. There was a feeling of being overwhelmed and little things were making her teary. Having been dwelling on the past, she now wanted to be involved in the present more. Also she was fearful for her mortality and she was jealous of others who were doing better financially.

Interestingly this time the remedies chosen with the exception of **Holly** and **Wild Rose** were all new choices. **Elm** for feeling overwhelmed, **Honeysuckle** for dwelling in the past, **Mustard** to deal with depression, **Rock Rose** for fear/terror, and **Willow** for resentment.

Case history summary

The main areas that Anne wanted to deal with were depression, family circumstances, and her irritable bladder. The remedies most used were **Beech** for intolerance, **Walnut** for protection of outside influences and, **Holly** for anger and jealousy. Although her bladder situation and depression, for the most part, remained, and she stayed on medication for these, I do believe that the emotional layers did begin to shift.

There were feelings of peace, and maybe she was working things out in her dreams. The last time I met with Anne she wanted to take **Mustard** to help deal with depression, and **Wild Rose** to assist with ambition, sense of purpose, and to make changes, bringing the spark back into her life.

I wish Anne well and hope that the remedies helped her on her journey to self and inner harmony healing.

Anne's testimonial - March 18, 2009

"I have many undiagnosed items with my health and started the Bach Flowers with the hope and anticipation that they may help in some way. I was not really sure what to expect for results.

I can say that I had a more calm feeling inside as the days went by. Interestingly I started having dreams every night for about 2 weeks - but what was interesting about this was they kept going further and further back in my life - reliving many different experiences I had gone through. None of which were bad but maybe somehow I needed to live them again. I don't know but I found it very fascinating.

I also had some mixture made up for my husband, who is so skeptical of taking these types of things. He did take the drops faithfully and I never referred to them. But near the end of the bottle he brought it up and said he felt much better psychologically.

I know that the drops are supposed to work insidiously so don't notice what changes take place. I do feel more centered and I do not dwell on what may happen like I used to. One of the main things I wanted to try them for was to cope with the addiction of my son. I think I don't dwell on his problems as I did - and realize it is his life and I cannot change his path - it's all up to him. I would like to think I am more balanced - I can't say I still don't have room to change but it is a start." **Anne**

What the Bach Flower Remedies can do for you...a reference chart

Flower Remedy	Negative Indication	Positive Indication
Agrimony	Hiding troubles behind humour.	Self-acceptance/inner joy.
Aspen	Vague, unknown fears, anxiety, terror or nightmares.	Trust in the unknown/fearlessness.
Beech	Intolerant and critical of others. Perfectionist.	Tolerance, and ability to see the good in others.
Centaury	Difficulty in saying "no" and easily led.	Assertiveness, ability to follow one's own path.
Cerato	Self-doubt and indecision. Seeking advice of others.	Confidence in one's own decisions.
Cherry Plum	Fear of losing control of mind, emotions, or body; suicidal tendencies, temper tantrums.	Mental calm and composure.
Chestnut Bud	Repetition of mistakes and inability to learn from them.	Ability to learn from mistakes and move forward.
Chicory	Over-concern for others; possessiveness.	Love and caring, with no strings attached.
Clematis	Daydreaming, lack of concentration in the present.	Being more grounded; having more interest in the here and now.

Flower Remedy	Negative Indication	Positive Indication
Crab Apple	Self-disgust, low self-esteem, and obsessed with cleanliness.	Positive self-image, and putting cleanliness into perspective.
Elm	Overwhelmed by many responsibilities.	Ability to put things into perspective. Self-assurance.
Gentian	Discouraged and despondent from setback of a known cause.	Encouragement and determination.
Gorse	Hopelessness, despair, and giving up hope.	Renewed hope.
Heather	Talkative lonely people, wanting to be the centre of attention.	Ability to be a good listener and have empathy.
Holly	Overcome by anger, jealousy, envy, and feelings of hatred.	Inner harmony; taking pleasure in the success of others.
Honeysuckle	Living in and dwelling on the past.	Involvement in the present.
Hornbeam	Procrastination and Monday-morning feeling.	Renewed energy and interest in life.
Impatiens	Impatient and irritated with the slow pace of others.	Patience.
Larch	Feeling inadequate and lacking self-confidence.	Confidence.

Flower Remedy	Negative Indication	Positive Indication
Mimulus	Fearful or anxious about something specific (known).	Bravery and courage.
Mustard	Baffling sadness, gloom and despair, like being under a black cloud.	Return of joy, inner stability and peace.
Oak	Having a sense of duty and struggling on despite exhaustion and against all odds.	Admitting limitations and taking time off to relax.
Olive	Mental and physical exhaustion.	Renewed subtle energy to get through the day.
Pine	Guilt and self-blame.	Self-respect and relief of guilty feelings.
Red Chestnut	Over-concern for the welfare of others (particularly loved ones) and fearing the worst.	Calm and rational concern.
Rock Rose	Extreme terror; fright, panic attacks, hysteria, etc.	Fearlessness; courage, calmness.
Rock Water	Strictness and self-denial.	Understanding and flexibility.
Scleranthus	Indecision and mood swings.	Decisive quick decisions with no dilemmas.
Star of Bethlehem	Distress and unhappiness following shock (timeless).	Comfort and consolation.

Flower Remedy	Negative Indication	Positive Indication
Sweet Chestnut	Anguish; those at the end of their endurance.	Optimism and peace of mind.
Vervain	Enthusiastic with fixed opinions and having an inability to relax.	Calm, tolerant, and able to unwind.
Vine	Dominant overbearing bossy leader.	Patient leader.
Walnut	Unable to break links with the past, and easily influenced.	Protection from change and outside influences. Able to move forward.
Water Violet	Proud and aloof. Although liking one's own company, sometimes feeling lonely.	Calm, serene, and more approachable.
White Chestnut	Obsessive and worrying thoughts that appear impossible to control.	Peace of mind and positive problem solving.
Wild Oat	Inability to find direction in life.	Purposefulness and decisive direction in life.
Wild Rose	Resignation, apathy, and disinterest in life.	Lively and enthusiastic interest in life.
Willow	Resentment, self-pity and bitterness.	Ability to forgive and forget. Back in control.

Photos taken in the Comox Valley by Sarah Brune

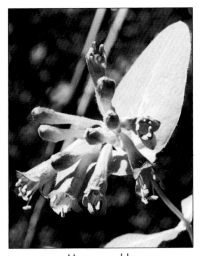

Honeysuckle

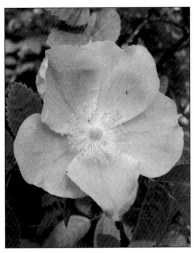

Wild Rose

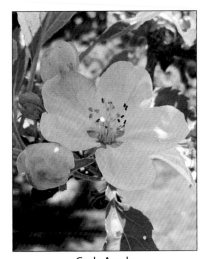

Crab Apple

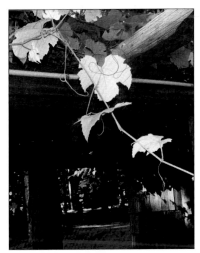

Vine

Photos taken in the Comox Valley by Sarah Brune

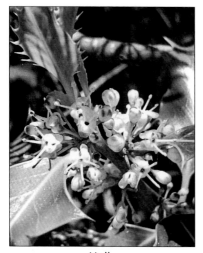

Holly

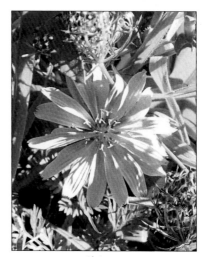

Chicory

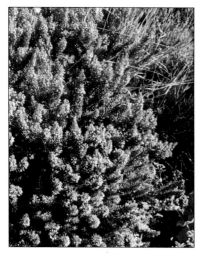

Heather

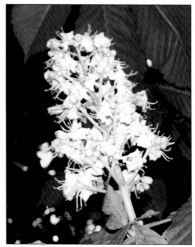

White Chestnut

Illustrations by Josie Brune

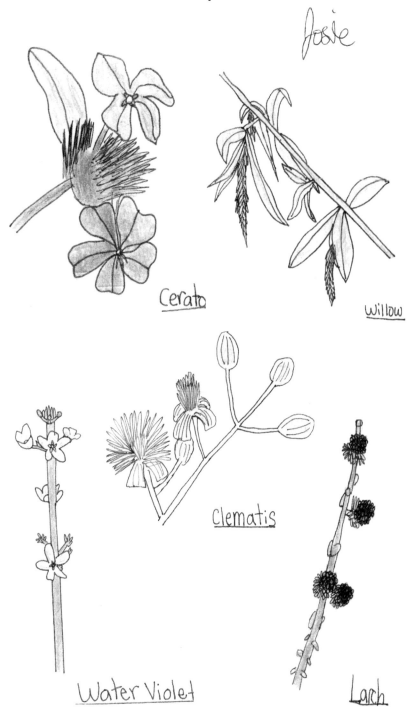

Josie

Cerato

Willow

Clematis

Water Violet

Larch

Illustrations by Josie Brune

Josie

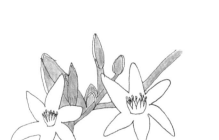

Star of Bethlehem

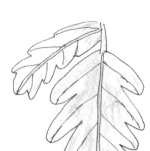

Oak

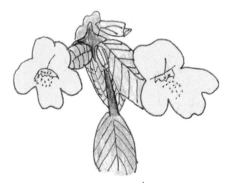

Mimulus

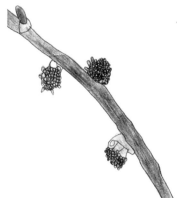

Elm

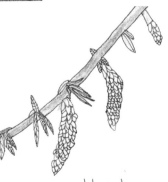

Hornbeam

The Bach Centre, Mt. Vernon, Oxfordshire, England

Photos taken by Sarah Brune©

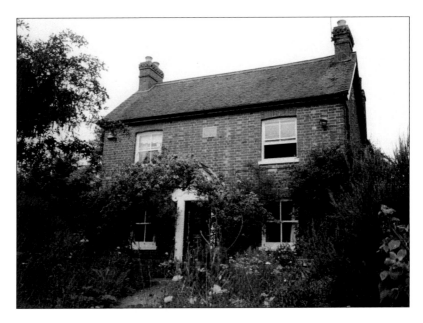

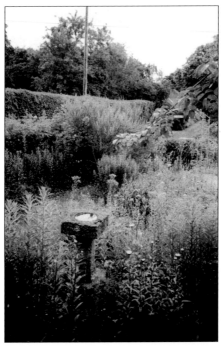

The Bach Centre, Mt. Vernon, Oxfordshire, England

Photos taken by Sarah Brune©

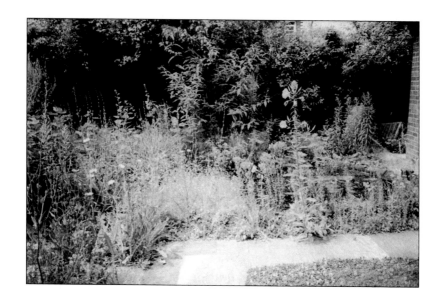

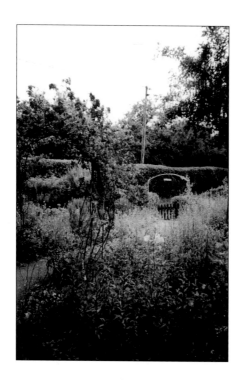

The Thirty-Eight Flower Remedies – some "reflections"

The flower remedies are set out with the negative indication, followed by the positive indication, and then the description of the remedy plant.

Agrimony
Agrimony eupatoria

Ah yes, they say with a laugh. All the way through the conversation they seem to joke around, always seeing things on the brighter side, even when the topic is not so great. They can be the life and soul of the party, and tend to live in the fast lane. I wish I could be that carefree. But, is their laughter genuine or a polite false laugh? You know the kind of short polite laugh that people use during a phone conversation or with someone they do not know very well?

Could it all be a charade of happiness, a mask used to disguise the turmoil that is really going on inside? Apart from cheerfulness, how do they manage to get through life – comfort food, alcohol, and drugs perhaps? Is the laughter actually painful, while inside they are crying?

After a few drops of Agrimony, they seem to be genuinely cheerful, and able to speak freely about their feelings. Their infectious smile makes you feel happy and brightens up your day.

The Agrimony plant looks like a giant yellow magic wand, maybe because it wishes to be something else, and with one wave everything is great and hunky-dory. The flowers on the long stalk take it in turns to come out into bloom three days each, as though they are lighting a taper of joy, from bottom to top.

Aspen

Populus tremula

After waking up with a start from a nightmare, hot and sweaty, there is a foreboding sense of uneasiness. What was all that about? I won't be able to get back to sleep now. Why am I so tense? Chills are going up and down my spine, my hands are trembling, and my heart is racing at 100 miles per hour. I don't know why I feel this way, but have a feeling something bad is going to happen. What, I do not know. I hate feeling like this! Please go away, fearful thoughts.

Sometimes life seems to present itself with worrying thoughts, out of nowhere, making my heart sink to my toes. The worst thing is, I cannot put my finger on it, but I know something bad is going to happen.

Thank you Aspen, for helping me get through this. I welcome the inner peace and tranquility. I am now ready for the world and whatever it may bring my way. No fear is too great. Bring it on!

The tall Aspen tree whispers in the wind as though it is trembling with fear, and consequently makes a spooky rustling sound. The leaves flutter in the slightest breeze as though to warn us that something bad is going to happen. The larger male and smaller female catkins grow on different trees and appear before the leaves. The catkins are soft and fluffy, just like a lamb's tail.

Beech

Fagus sylvatica

The neatly dressed lady was having a drink in the coffee shop, while she looked around disapprovingly at the other two patrons. Unimpressed, she decided to refrain from going there again. An elderly man sat huddled next to the fireplace and a woman sat directly opposite her. The elderly man's thinning hair, in her opinion, was too long, and could do with a decent haircut. His dry flaking skin would benefit from some moisturizer, and for the reddish complexion, she was at a loss for ideas. What shocked her most was what he was wearing; an old shabby lumberjack shirt, paint stained jeans, and tatty shoes that had seen better days.

The woman opposite her slouched over her coffee and instantly met with her disapproval. Her casual attire of loosely fitting sweat pants and sweatshirt did not suit her one bit. The outfit did not go well with her cheap-looking purse and shabby black shoes. Due to an obvious weight problem she should refrain from eating such rich food.

After taking some Beech, she realized that her views of them had been rather harsh after all. Perhaps the elderly man had a hard life working outside and he was short on cash. Maybe he was just having a break from work, hence the casual attire. The woman may have just been to the gym and felt as though she deserved a nice currant bun after her hard workout.

The tall Beech tree with silver grey bark is decorated with light seaweed-green leaves. Dangling from the branches on long stems are odd-looking flowers that are green/white with tinges of pink. It is as though someone is trying to make pompom curtain tassels out of green, white, and pink wool.

Centaury
Centaurium umbellatum

Yes, sure, no problem. I am happy to help. I like being able to help out whenever needed, no matter how tired I am. Once I have picked up their kids and mine from school, I will nip over to an elderly friend's place and do a bit of cleaning for them. (They asked so nicely I couldn't say "no.") After that, I will make supper for everyone, take the kids to sports practice, and then take everyone home again.

Of course the kids can stay over, no problem. You are busy, and I would love to take your dog for a walk and of course he can stay over too. It'll be fun. Oh no, it's no trouble at all. I must admit by the end of the day after being the Good Samaritan I feel absolutely exhausted, and I never get any time to myself.

Now that I have had some Centaury and had time to think, I suppose that people were beginning to take advantage of my good nature. But no more. Today I am going to do what I want to do! It's time to draw the line and only help when absolutely necessary. In fact, I am going to the spa so I can be pampered for a change.

Centaury is an attractive plant with small, rose-pink, star-like flowers. The plant seems a bit top-heavy with a mass of flowers at the top of the stem, as though it is dressed to impress. The second part of the Latin name, umbellatum, makes me think that perhaps the flowers at the top of the stem act as an umbrella, keeping everyone dry at their own expense.

Cerato

Ceratostigma willmottiana

I can't decide if I should go and work out of the new store or not. My other dilemma is that they want me to sign a binding contract. Something doesn't feel quite right. Oh, what to do? I've just had a brilliant idea. I'll ask as many people as I know what they think I should do, and then I will come to my final decision.

After asking everyone's opinion, I am more confused than ever and my head is spinning. What is wrong with me? Why can't I make a decision? Maybe I should do some more research, write down the pros and cons and then make my decision.

Thanks Cerato for my epiphany, and I now know what to do after all. Deep down I knew what I wanted to do and just confused myself by asking everyone else's opinions. I will go with my gut feeling and keep things as they were.

The deep blue/purple flowers of the Cerato plant are a decisive, distinct colour. The five petals are delicate, and towards the centre they turn white, as though they are looking inward for their inner wisdom and the light at the end of the tunnel.

Cherry Plum
Prunus cerasifera

I feel as though I am on the verge of a volcanic eruption of anger, and once I start to yell, there is no stopping me. I may sound calm, but believe me, I am not. If I were a child I would be having a major temper tantrum and throwing myself on the floor kicking and screaming and yelling with rage, with the feeling that nobody understands why I am so mad. It's not that I like feeling this way, and I do sometimes feel fearful of losing control of my emotions, or my sanity for that matter.

Thank you Cherry Plum, I feel calmer now, and at last can think with a rational mind. I no longer feel as though I am going to lose it. I am now more composed and better at controlling my temper.

The Cherry Plum blossom is pure white, and resembles delicate rice paper or confetti. In between the five petals are numerous protruding stamens, similar to the sparks coming from a sparkler. In full blossom, the tree brings a splash of white and an air of beauty to the spring day.

Chestnut Bud
Aesculus hippocastanum

After a long hard day of work, I look forward to a relaxing evening and some time for myself. We eat at 6 p.m., and afterwards take the dogs for a walk. Then, after putting on my night attire I can hear the couch calling my name.

After a while during the commercials I go into the kitchen to make myself a cup of tea and go to the "junk" cupboard to see what can alleviate my "snack attack." After a bowl of chips, I feel like having something sweet. A cookie helps, but then I remember the chocolate bar that looked rather lonely on the top shelf.

Half an hour later, I complain to my husband that I have eaten too much and feel sick! Oh yes! His reply is always the same, "It's your own fault for eating so much," but I always seem to forget. For some reason I always get into a rut, and never learn from my mistakes.

Chestnut Bud helps me to realize that enough is enough. Next time I go grocery shopping I am not going to buy any "junk food." Another solution is to see if there are any clubs or classes worth joining, to keep me busy and off the couch.

The Chestnut Bud grows next to the scars of last year's leaves and tightly hangs onto how things were. Gradually it opens up to hopes and dreams, spreading its leaves out to a new, fresh, clean start.

Chicory
Chichorium intybus

Oh, Chicory, how you remind us of our mothers, who want the best for their children, but on their terms. But alas, why do our mothers sometimes go too far and want to control our lives? Interfering, nagging, critical, they have the amazing ability to make us feel guilty. Why are you so contrary? Is it really necessary? In fact, there are times when I do not enjoy your company or phone call, and come away feeling depressed. I refuse to be influenced by your negative ways.

Ah, at last you have taken a sip of Chicory. You have seen the light and want us to be happy with the lifestyle we choose. Your unselfish love, understanding, and encouragement is welcome and you are a thoughtful loving mother again. I must admit it seems strange receiving compliments from you, and having a pleasant conversation, after all these years. What a surreal experience.

What a beautiful light blue flower with long thin petals. Long green, waxy stems, tall and thin, each flower taking its turn to be in full bloom. Chicory, I was looking for you. I knew you were there, but you were hiding low down in the grass amongst the dandelions. Your attractive light mauve/blue flower caught my eye and reminded me of soft feathers. In the centre of the flower the blue stamens stand out and resemble sparkling flames coming out of a sparkler.

Clematis
Clematis vitalba

Sorry. What did you say? I was miles and miles away; in Hawaii to be exact, basking in the sunshine. Those warm rays feel so good on my face. It is so blissful walking along the beach in the soft sand, hearing the waves lap against the shore. Oh, yes, sorry, my mind is just not with it today. Hold on a minute, I just need to check my email, and then I am all ears.

You see I yearn for better times. Life is boring, so I just like to escape into my own imaginary world where life is good, as it helps me to ignore reality. I can't be bothered with trying to change things. There is no point and besides it will do no good. I think I will go out on the yacht now that I have moored off my private island in Hawaii.

Clematis you have given me an epiphany. Maybe I should try to concentrate and finish writing this book, and see what I can do to make life better and more fulfilling. I have just come back down to earth with a bang, and if things go according to plan, in a year or so Hawaii may become a reality and not just a daydream. It is just a matter of focusing on the here and now, and making things happen. Better go and get myself sorted out and have a realistic plan of action.

Clematis an airy-fairy looking plant that is all over the place, climbing over hedges and banks from June to September. Its green-white flowers smell of vanilla. Then in the fall they change to attractive fluffy seed heads with silvery grey thread-like tails that look like an old man's beard.

Crab Apple
Malus pumila

I just can't seem to get the house clean, despite scrubbing it from top to bottom. It has taken me hours to get everything sanitary, but however hard I try, it still looks dirty. You would not think that I go through this ritual every day.

Another thing that is bothering me right now is my hair. Despite my best efforts, every day seems to be a "bad hair" day.

The fact that I wash it several times a day does not seem to help in the slightest. I cannot possibly go out in public looking like this. If, and when, I do go out, I put on my smartest clothes, wear lots of makeup to hide my awful complexion, and I wear a hat.

Crab Apple, thank you for helping me to put things in perspective. I don't know why I worry about my complexion, it only has a few blemishes, and nobody else would be able to see them without a magnifying glass. The house is not that bad; I guess I have been going a bit over the top with cleaning. I am just going to chill out and relax for a while in my nice clean house.

The blossoms on the Crab Apple look fresh and clean, like freshly washed sheets hanging on the line. The white flowers are tinted with pink, and the petals are heart shaped.

Elm

Ulmus procera

How on earth can I get everything done in such a short time? I don't think I can cope; in fact, it is all making me feel anxious and depressed. Company is coming tomorrow, and I need to tidy the whole house, do the shopping, prepare a menu and cook some meals in advance, get the bill payments up to date, and so it goes on. Ah, it is all too much. I just don't know where to start.

I know if I sit down with a cup of tea and I drop some Elm in it, maybe things won't look so bad. To start things off I will make a list of what's to be done, and then I'll prioritize the list. I will get the kids to help with some of the housework, then if someone gets the groceries that will help. The rest I can do in no time. I don't know what I was thinking; the house does not need to be that perfect, just slightly neat and tidy. Nobody is going to do the white glove test for dust. Then this evening I can catch up with any other work that needs doing, like paying the bills. Sometimes I just panic, and I know deep down that I am capable of doing things.

In the spring, the branches of the Elm tree have clusters of round reddish purple/ brown buds, which from a distance resemble delicious toffee apples. They later turn into leaves.

Gentian
Gentiana amarella

What a day! Nothing seems to be going right and that job rejection did not help either. Disappointment is setting in. It's very much like having a slap in the face with a bungee chord that has snapped loose, and it is stinging like crazy. I guess I should not have pinned my hopes on passing that exam or getting that job. To cap it all, the dog has injured its leg again, and the last straw is that the computer is on the blink again. Rejection and things going wrong do not sit well with me. In fact, I am feeling so depressed and discouraged that, until further notice, I will lie on the couch hiding under a blanket from the cruel, unfair world.

Thank you, Gentian for helping me to feel so much better. I am just not going to let anything get to me. These minor bumps in the road have to be taken face on, and I am strong enough to be able to cope with things. It is time to get off the couch. My plan of action is to take care of the dog as best as I can, look for another job, and get the computer fixed. Next time the exam results are due, I will take some Gentian just to be on the safe side. My new motto is onward and upward.

The star-shaped Gentian flower is a distinctive purple/blue, so it is going to be my star of hope and encouragement. A superstar.

Gorse
Ulex europaeus

What's the point! It is hopeless! Things will never improve. I might as well get used to it. Things are obviously destined to be this way. When others try to encourage me to do things there just does not seem to be much point. I may try another treatment or try for another job, but I doubt if it will do any good or make things better.

Ah, Gorse you have been so supportive and I feel alive again. You have brought some sunshine and hope into my life. I can now see the light at the end of the tunnel. The clouds of doom are burning off and from now on I will look on the brighter side of life. I'll try to live by the words from the ending song in the Life of Brian, "Always look on the bright side of life."

Gorse flowers are bright yellow like a beautiful golden sun shining brightly in the sky. I will try to imagine them on the next cold, damp, depressing, foggy day and let the Gorse's golden sun take me back to the days of my youth when I was lying on a sandy beach on a Greek island soaking up the sun and then cooling down by diving into the ocean.

Heather

Calluna vulgaris

Chitter-chatter, chitter-chatter; surely, everyone is interested in my latest ailment. I must make sure to tell them in as much detail as possible how the phlegm drips down the back of my throat when I feel a cold coming on. It is also necessary to tell them in as much detail as possible about my journey to their house, for instance how many sets of red traffic lights I encountered, or what happened on the train journey. It is all so fascinating, and so nice to be in the company of others, as I do get lonely at home all on my own.

Do you want to know a really good way of preventing people from leaving early? Stand in front of the door and put your arm across it. Works every time! Of course, the conversation always revolves around me.

A drop or two of Heather and hey, presto – a compassionate person who is interested in others, and being a good listener, yes that's right actually listening to others for a change. Not someone that people want to avoid, but someone they genuinely want to strike up a conversation with. Others are pleasantly surprised that they are so empathetic, and come away feeling better about things.

Heather, a pretty purple plant bringing some colour to scrublands, moors, and barren areas. The rough and wiry stems are covered with an array of flowers that look like bells. The overall effect is a carpet of purple and green than can be seen for miles and miles, as though it wants to be the centre of attention.

Holly

Ilex aquifolium

It's not fair. Why did they get the larger room, more frequent visits, numerous holidays, and fancy vehicles? Not that I am jealous, you understand, but I cannot bear rich people these days. I know this sounds awful, but I hope something bad happens to them. It will serve them right for being so high and mighty, and thinking they are so wonderful. Since they have become more affluent they seem to have changed, and not for the good, in my opinion. I feel like screaming from the rooftops at them. I am not in the slightest bit interested in their successes, or take any interest in their lives, as they are far too pompous. After all, who cares?

Holly has helped me open up my heart and to see things from a more compassionate outlook. I now realize they have worked hard and had a certain number of sacrifices to make. Good for them. One must live and let live, and be happy for those around us.

The white and pinkish flowers on the Holly are so delicate, yet surrounded by spiked, prickly leaves that turn into plump, red berries. The plant's makeup is very much like the Holly person, who has prickly outer layers, but can be compassionate and have a soft heart. The Holly bush brings colour to the yard over the winter months, and although the berries are poisonous to people, they provide food for the birds.

Honeysuckle

Lonicera caprifolium

Oh, for the good old days, so much fun, adventure, and good times. That's all in the past now with only the odd photo of how things used to be. Life just seemed so much simpler and carefree back then. I guess it was because I was young, footloose, and fancy-free. Staying out all night partying and drinking pink champagne, coming home late on the night bus. Best of all I could be unreliable, irresponsible, and devious.

As a child, I remember trying to suck the honey out of the honeysuckle flowers growing in our garden. It is like the sweet sorrow memories of the past. I feel sad that it is all gone. I guess Christmas brings back memories of Christmases gone by, and how the whole day seemed such a special occasion with a set menu and timetable. Oh, for just one more Christmas at home, presents after the Queen's speech at three, the party poppers, crackers, bread sauce, and "flaming" Christmas pudding.

After taking a sip of Honeysuckle I gradually began thinking more about the future and using what was learned from the past. Time moves on and so does life with families and responsibilities. So much for being unreliable and irresponsible. As far as being devious is concerned, I can hardly stay awake after 11:00 p.m., darn it. Fortunately, there are opportunities out there and other good times that suit my age; going to the theatre instead of a wine bar and holidaying in Hawaii and staying in a fancy hotel, rather than sleeping on the beach.

The Honeysuckle flower resembles delicate fairies with full ballet dresses dancing around in circles with their thin, whispery legs. Their dresses are made from the finest yellow silk that compliments their light or dark pink wings.

Hornbeam

Carpinus betulus

I could not be bothered to get out of bed today, period. I am comfortable, warm and cozy, plus it is snowing outside. There is nothing much to do today anyway. Just five more minutes.

Getting out of bed and gradually going downstairs, it feels as though I am dragging a big lead weight behind me. Okay, I am up. Now what? Oh, no. I wish I had done the dishes last night. Never mind. They can wait. Instead, I will go and play with the dogs outside in the snow.

Company is coming. Quick let's take some Hornbeam so I can get all that boring housework out of the way. That was not too bad. I managed to get it all done in the end, and it did not take very long to do. The dark, misty fog of procrastination did not take long to lift and now life seems brighter and more fun.

The many male and female catkins grow on the same tree and appear similar to long braids of dirty blonde hair hanging off the branches. Each braid is intermingled with light green, pointed leaves.

Impatiens
Impatiens glandulifera

Hurry up. I can't wait all day you know. We all have families to go home to. You don't seem to realize, but this has to be done right away. For goodness sake let me do it. You go home and I will do it myself. Honestly, some people just do not seem to get with the program. Time is money and it is such a simple task. If they worked any slower, they would stop. I just want to get going at this new venture. Why do some things take so long to happen? Patience is meant to be a virtue, but sorry, no can do.

After taking some Impatiens I now realize the saying "Rome was not built in a day" rings true. I suppose they were doing their best and taking their time to do the job properly. From now on, I will get less stressed about deadlines, as it is not doing my blood pressure any good. It is not the "be all and end all." I will sit back and enjoy my coffee while reading the paper.

What was that, Impatiens? You look as though you are trying to tell me something. I only said that because your pale crimson petals are shaped like a lip and mouth. All right, all right. I will hurry up and carry on with my walk.

Larch

Larix decidua

I don't know if I will be able to do that. I am not very good at public speaking, and will probably blush. I don't do well in exams, and do not usually get good marks at school. I want to get on in life and succeed, but do not think it is possible. Why even try?

After a few drops of Larch, I feel a bit more positive about life, and will try my hand at doing things I was not willing to try before. Why sit at home twiddling my thumbs when there is so much out there in the world that I have never thought I could do before? You will never know until you try. My wise Grandmother always used to say, "There is no such word as can't." How true.

Male and female catkins grow on the same tree on drooping twigs, coming out into bloom just as the leaves are appearing. The male catkins are golden yellow, and of course totally outshone by the bright red round female's blooming catkins. The red is spectacular. Brighter than fire engine red. Almost florescent.

Mimulus

Mimulus guttatus

The alarm went off, and she woke up with a start. Oh no, today is the day of my presentation, she thought and her heart sank to her toes. It was the day that she had been dreading for months; so many fearful thoughts were preying on her mind.

It was not just the presentation. Having to fly to the conference centre was her worst fear. What if she missed her flight? Was the weather too bad for the plane to take off? Would the plane crash? Would she forget to take her laptop? Worse still, would it work? Was her outfit smart enough, and would it crease on the journey? What happened if she went bright red? Would there be a large audience? She did not like speaking in public. Oh no, how would she get through the day?

While drinking her coffee (laced with Mimulus), she tried to reassure herself that all would be well. Her laptop was in good working order and she had practiced her speech over many a time. Besides, the conference centre had a copy of her notes there. It was a bright sunny day and she had checked that her flight was on schedule. Later that evening, after the day went without a "hitch" she could not understand what she had been so fearful of, and could not wait until her next presentation.

The bright yellow wild Mimulus grows by streams and brooks in the English countryside. The perfect petals look as if they have been delicately painted with reddish spots, perhaps to attract insects. The colour reminds me of my childhood bedroom that I so wanted to be painted bright, cheery, primrose yellow.

Mustard

Sinapis arvensis

Sometimes life is just all doom and gloom, and there does not seem to be any reason to be happy. Things may be going well, but it does not make me feel any better. It is as though I am being followed around by a big dark rain cloud. One minute everything seems fine, and then unexpectedly out of nowhere, this wretched, dark, damp cloud of depression engulfs me and I am unable to shake it off.

All the life and joy has been sucked out of me, as if I have been attacked by a Dementore from one of the Harry Potter books. It makes me feel cold, withered, and old, with every ounce of happiness gone. It is a forgotten entity to feel happy and contented. It is all doom and gloom, and sadly, it is for no apparent reason.

At last after taking some Mustard, the dark gray clouds have parted and I see blue sky and sunlight again. A sense of peace and inner harmony has returned, after a long rainstorm. Things seem better and life returns to normal. Nothing can ruffle my feathers now.

This invasive bushy plant grows in fields and waysides, producing many pods to reproduce easily. The bright yellow flowers grow in numerous clusters. It's as though the bright yellow flowers want to spread cheer and happiness to all who walk by.

Oak
Quercus robur

Solid reliable Oak, plodding along slowly at whatever you are doing and not stopping until the task is done. Even when things seem hopeless, you carry on regardless of failure. Why do you try so hard, and hit your head against a wall? Isn't it wearing you down being a strong pillar of strength? Life does not have to be taken so seriously. Why don't you sit down and relax, and go and have some fun? You have amazing stamina, but please do not be too hard on yourself.

Here dear, take a drop of Oak. Ah yes, that is better. We should go out tonight and have some fun! Let's be spontaneous, wild and crazy, he says singing a joyful tune (to the annoyance of the children). First let's sit and relax and look out of the window at the freshly cut lawn, and not be bothered about cleaning the dirty windows.

As I sit under the mighty Oak tree that has stood firm for hundreds of years, I look up and admire how the thick trunk supports so many branches, which are covered with numerous leaves. It seems that it has a sense of duty to provide me with so much shade.

Olive
Olea europaea

My get up and go, just got up and went. I feel so tired and exhausted, and cannot seem to shake off this annoying cold. Even the thought of cooking the meal or going upstairs makes me feel tired. In fact, another nap is in order and most probably an early night again. I am sick and tired of feeling sick and tired! Everything seems to be like hard work these days, and I feel as if a large weight is attached to my feet, slowing me down. Even the thought of rest and relaxation is tiring.

Goodness! After only a few drops of Olive I have managed to get a lot done today: the laundry, the house cleaning, and some yard work. That was just the tip of the iceberg, but better than nothing. I seem to have regained my energy without noticing it. The spring has returned to my step.

Hidden amongst the grey-green feather-shaped leaves of the olive tree are inconspicuous cream fragrant flowers. It is as if there is a subtle reserve of energy lurking and waiting until we need it.

Pine

Pinus sylvestris

Guilt, guilt, and more guilt. Why do I always feel so guilty about leaving the dogs alone when I go out? Sometimes it is hard to enjoy myself thinking of them being cooped up inside. Mind you, if I had been paying more attention while the dogs were playing outside Harry would not have injured his leg in the first place and have to spend most his time inside. Even when I am sick and don't have the energy to do anything, I feel guilty about lying in bed. I even apologize to the family and dogs for not being able to get out of bed.

After taking a sip of Pine, the penny has dropped and I have finally freed myself from a life of guilt. Life is so much more enjoyable. My dogs may be cute and cuddly and have big brown eyes, but they cannot tell the time. Harry's leg is getting better by the day. They are still happy to see me when I return and love me unconditionally. I am not indispensable and everyone else is perfectly capable of helping around the house when I am sick. What a relief not having to look at my watch all the time, and not feeling so guilty about everything. Let's go party!

The mighty slender pine trees stand firm in our yard. They drop pine needle after pine needle, as though leaving a trail to remind us we are needed at home, and how dare we go out.

Red Chestnut
Aesculus carnea

I'm thinking of the worst, and every scenario that can go wrong; an accident, a bully, a robbery, or a fire ... I want my family to be safe at all times and hope that nothing bad happens to them.

I hear a yelp from the yard, and my dog Harry starts to limp badly. Oh no. Tears roll down my cheeks. Quick! Call the vet. I'm trying to comfort my dog while feeling so helpless and trying to imagine the pain he is suffering. Practically in hysterics I talk to friends on the phone. They offer to meet me at the vet's.

Wondering how the children will take the bad news, and I hope to be back in time to pick them up from school. Cautiously I help Harry into the vehicle, and take large sips of Red Chestnut all the way to the vet's.

Worried about a loved one, never fear Red Chestnut is here. It gives us the strength to remain calm and the knowledge that things will work out all right in the end. It is possible to be a pillar of strength for the dog and children and you will be there when needed, at last feeling better and knowing that help is close to hand. He will get better and I have a long rehab job ahead of me. Everything will be fine, and there is no need to worry.

The striking Red Chestnut flower, reminds me of a large distinctive torch – shining and giving a glimmer of hope and reassurance that help is near at hand and all will be well.

Rock Rose
Helianthemum nummularium

My hands were trembling, my heart was thumping away, I was nervous, and my stomach was in knots. Not being able to move, a total numbness had overcome me. I was frozen to the spot and my mouth was as dry as a bone. I was experiencing an overbearing feeling of terror. I just sat there while being beaten, not able to scream nor defend myself, let alone fight back. There was such a mean look in their eyes, and it was as though they were taking pleasure in beating me with their belt. It was as if they had cast a spell on me to make me feel and act that way.

Wow, what an awful memory. It still haunts my dreams from time to time. Thank you Rock Rose, from relieving me of those feelings, helping me to feel calmer and more courageous. I will carry you around with me to help others whenever they seem to be in need, after an accident, or assault, and giving them the strength to get over it.

Delicate buttercup yellow Rock Rose, you look so flimsy and crumpled, but provide us with so much strength and reassurance. The splash of colour you provide is a carpet of courage.

Rock Water

Aqua petra

I like to work hard, and not over-indulge in the pleasures of life. As far as food is concerned I eat to live, and try to avoid desserts at all costs. My clothes are plain. My shirt or blouse or cardigan is always buttoned all the way up. Under no circumstances do I want to bring attention to myself. As for makeup, only when I am older, perhaps? My day consists of getting up early and practicing the piano, followed by a long run. Meals are a necessity and no great effort should be made with preparing them. I work hard at school and always do my homework as soon as I get home. The evenings are spent reading, watching a documentary or the news on TV.

I try my hardest at everything I do, and like to do well in life. My aspirations are to get a top-notch job and to be affluent. All right, I do have high ideals, but failure is unacceptable. One tries to set a good example to others.

All right then (she says after a sip of Rock Water), maybe I will have that piece of strawberry ice cream cake, be a devil and let my hair down, literally (normally it is tied in a tight ponytail).

That bright purple skirt I saw at the store is a possibility for the party that I will go to after all. My gray skirt can be left for more formal occasions such as interviews. Generally, my mind will be changed about certain things if I really believe that it is the right thing to do, but it is necessary to set a good example to others.

Stone cold, spring rock water to be found in secluded areas in its natural form, partly, in view of the sun, and partly shaded by trees.

Scleranthus

Scleranthus annuus

"I can't decide which dress to wear today mum," the indecisive child whines to her mother. The clock is ticking and it's not long before school starts. The mother delicately tries to negotiate with her child to please choose either the blue or the red dress as quickly as possible. Eventually after a long teary scene and raised voices, the child puts on the blue dress. The mother is absolutely exhausted.

Decisions do not come easily for the child and life is so full of decisions – she is so confused by the choices and decisions that it makes her head spin. As if that was not bad enough, she feels happy one minute and sad the next.

After taking some Scleranthus, the "knots" of confusion and indecision gradually untangle. Clear sudden decisive thoughts enter the child's mind from nowhere. Why hadn't she thought of that before? Life is so much more balanced and straightforward now. Much to the relief of her mother, the young child decides in a flash, which dress to wear.

The Scleranthus plant is comparable to a tangled piece of wool. At random, the tangled stems produce spiked, waxy green flowers, which grow in all directions.

Star of Bethlehem

Ornithogalum umbellatum

Fiona was in a car accident five years ago. Her whiplash was getting better, but the emotional wounds had not yet started healing. It had all happened so quickly. One minute she had been in the car with her fiancé, happy and without a care in the world, and the next, a vehicle appeared from nowhere and her fiancé was hunched up over the steering wheel dead. There was a feeling of loss, grief, sadness, and numbness. Nothing seemed to help her get over the shock and trauma.

Wow, thank you Star of Bethlehem, I feel so much better now. My emotional wounds are gradually healing over time and will soon be faded scars. The memory of the terrible events is being pushed further and further to the back of my mind. The remedies, counseling, and physiotherapy have done their part helping her whiplash and emotional pain. Star of Bethlehem you were my savior neutralizing the pain of what happened.

Thank goodness for Star of Bethlehem, a delicate white star-shaped flower, being the comforter and soother of pains and sorrows. It is a star of hope reaching out to us in our time of need and assisting to neutralize the negative feelings.

Sweet Chestnut

Castanea sativa

Ever since childhood, all the young girl ever wanted and yearned for was to be a wife and mother. In her early thirties, the young woman married. As her husband was often away for long periods, there was not much progress on the "baby front."

Nearing her mid-thirties, the young woman was getting concerned about no baby being in sight and her "clock was ticking." Due to trouble conceiving, fertility treatment was suggested. Now in her late thirties and after several failed fertility treatments the woman began to think that she would never have children. The more she thought about being childless, the more obsessed and depressed she became.

Nearing 40, she feared that her childhood dream of

becoming a mother was squashed. Despite suggestions and encouragement from others, she turned a deaf ear and wanted to close the case on becoming a mother. She cried and sobbed day and night. Hopelessness prevailed. The only thing that would make her happy would be to have a baby. She was engulfed in deep anguish and total despair.

After taking some Sweet Chestnut, the depression and anguish gradually lifted and slowly but surely after many months she became less obsessed with having a baby. She took a livelier interest in life and tried to keep herself busy volunteering. The 40-year-old woman decided to try to let it go and perhaps there may be a tiny glimmer of hope that she would one day be a mother.

The droopy, dark green leaves on the Sweet Chestnut tree look so sad. It is as though they make no effort to be happy. Then suddenly caterpillar-like flowers appear which are fragrant and sticky and produce a sweet fruit.

Vervain
Verbena officinalis

The speaker had been very convincing and enthusiastic about his particular product, and spoke with a loud booming voice. He was anxious to get his point of view across to the audience that they should all sign on the dotted line today.

He had done a good job because over half of those in the audience did sign up, but others were not entirely convinced. The speaker went around trying to convince them about his wonderful product. He was not willing to take "no" for an answer. After a lot of coaxing, some more people signed up, and those who did not were coaxed further. The speaker was pleased with the outcome, and as people left he said, "Please remember it is now up to you, to spread the word and convince everyone else to buy this wonderful product."

Excitable over-enthusiastic Vervain, keyed up, with their own strict agenda and views, who seem to be always on the go. Are you able to relax or sleep at night?

Wow! What a totally different person you are after taking a few drops of Vervain. You are calm, relaxed, tolerant and patient, and so much easier going. I can actually have a decent conversation with you now, and not feel so pressured to do as you ask.

Vervain is a tall straggly plant that seems to be all over the place, each stalk going in a different direction. At the tip of each stalk, delicate lilac flowers grow. The lower buds open and flower first.

Vine

Vitis vinifera

His decision was closed-minded. "It is my way or the highway," he said in a loud, domineering voice to the few hangers-on. "I am innocent, so let's get rid of those who are ganging up on me. I can assure you it is the right thing to do and everyone will benefit, just you wait and see. Nobody is going to get in my way. If necessary, I will make life miserable for those who do not see things from my point of view. Then they had better change their minds."

"Let's get everyone together to try and see if we can work things out for the better," he said after having a sip of Vine. "Everyone will have a chance to let his or her views be known. Our long-term objective is to make everyone happy and work as a team."

The Vine plant lets nothing get in its way, grasping on, suffocating and choking everything in its path. It is a long-lived climbing plant with woody stems, producing sweet grapes.

Walnut

Juglans regia

But I don't like change. Why do we have to grow old and endure physical changes? I like being young and wrinkle free. If that's not bad enough, when I get an idea in my head about something like going off traveling, like clockwork someone always tries to talk me out of it and ruins everything. On second thoughts, maybe they do have a point. I am confused now.

Life is full of changes as friends come and go. They either move away or get into bad habits, and I am left all alone. Everything was going so well.

Walnut, thank goodness for Walnut. It is the protector from change, distraction, and influences. It helps keep us on the straight and narrow path. Change can be upsetting, and Walnut can assist by moving us on with confidence, as well as giving us the ability to walk away unscathed, without looking back.

The big bold Walnut tree has twisted branches that make an upward turn, assisting us through the unpredictable twists and turns of life. Inside its hard shell it protects us from change and criticism.

Water Violet

Hottonia palustris

One minute she is locked away in her 'Ivory Tower' shutting out and protecting herself from the outside world, appearing aloof. Then gradually and slowly, she comes out appearing delicate, quiet, and calm, never wanting to be disturbed, criticized, or in the limelight. Often she keeps her troubles to herself and secludes herself from others.

She is the councillor and advisor. She does not want to interfere, but is always there to help others when needed. She works hard in the background and does great things. The Water Violet's peace and calmness is noticed everywhere she goes. She goes through life treading gracefully, like a young child skipping through a meadow of wild flowers, stopping to admire the flowers as she floats by.

Gentle, delicate Water Violet stands upright and alone partly submerged in water. The fragile pale lilac flowers grow in clusters of five hanging onto the long stem above the water, while the leaves are sunken below the water. The flowers resemble flowing chiffon dresses that young ballerinas might wear to perform in a ballet, as they gently dance across the stage like a breath of fresh air.

White Chestnut

Aesculus hippocastanum

I just cannot concentrate today because these wretched thoughts keep going around and around in my head. Decisions, decisions. That is the problem. Shall I or shan't I? It is not too bad during the day, but at night when I am trying to get to sleep, the thoughts spinning in my head escalate as if they are an out-of-control merry-go-round. Sometimes the thoughts fill me with worry about things that have to be done, or some big decision, and my thoughts drive me crazy.

Ah, at last some peace and tranquility – thank you White Chestnut. Everything seems crystal clear now and I can focus on what needs to be done. Why worry? Things all seem to work out for the best. As an added bonus, I can look forward to a more restful sleep.

The mighty White Chestnut has flowers that together resemble a white beacon of light watching over us while we sleep soundly.

Wild Oat

Bromus ramosus

It's time for another adventure. I am getting itchy feet, and I am bored with this dead-end job. There is a whole world out there that needs to be explored, interesting places to visit, another mountain to climb, and maybe I could combine my trip with voluntary work. Oh, to be free again, nobody telling me what to do, free as a kite blowing in the wind. Maybe one day I will figure out what I really want to do with my life. It is on the tip of my tongue. In the mean time, I will stick a pin in a map, and off I will go until something more interesting comes along.

At last, it has come to me; I know exactly what I want to do. Thank you, Wild Oat. The funny thing is, it was staring me in the face all along. Without knowing it, I wrote down where I wanted to live in a friend's visitors book, and the move actually materialized. Wow, I am actually happy now living on a beautiful island, working and having found the man of my dreams.

Straggly looking Wild Oat grows in hedgerows and wooded areas, and by the roadside, helping those lost to find their way. Tall thin grass with a drooping head, it scatters its seeds wherever the wind takes them.

Wild Rose
Rosa canina

Life is stale and boring. There is no point trying to make an effort anymore. It is no use. My get-up-and go, got up and went. Being stuck in a rut is not so bad once you get used to it. I will just "ride out the waves" and put up with things. You never know. Things might change with time.

Today, after taking some Wild Rose, I'm on top of the world, feeling refreshed and recharged like a jump started dead car battery. It's time to get out there and see what opportunities are lurking around the corner. Farewell, stale boring life. Hello, world. I am back and rearing to go. Isn't life fantastic?

The beautiful Wild English Rose carries a sweet smell to those walking by. Such a subtle shade of powder pink, it looks so gentle, yet the plant is hardy.

Willow
Salix vitellina

It is not fair! Why do they get to do fun things and go to exciting places, while I am stuck here at boring old home? To make it worse the weather is awful and even if I wanted to I could not go anywhere, not that there is anywhere of interest to go anyway. I cannot bear rich happy people. They probably do not appreciate the simpler things in life. Well, I feel sorry for myself even if no one else does. Others just do not seem to get it, and need to get with the program. I am stuck in a rut and nothing or no one can change that.

You know what? Life is not that bad (after taking a drop or two of Willow); maybe there is light at the end of the tunnel after all. I guess all this negativity has been preventing good things from happening. In a way, we have to be in control of our lives, be open to our destiny, generally enjoy life and what it brings.

The male and female catkins grow on different trees and are primarily pollinated by the wind. The catkins droop downwards and are enveloped by long pointed leaves. They remind me of a green upside down banana. They look limp and sad as though they could not be bothered to do much.

Life's Reflections

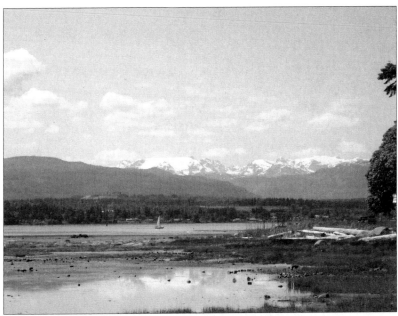

Glacier in the Comox Valley, BC

Sometimes day-to-day events or life in general do not go according to plan. Whether it is making preparations or arrangements for a particular vocation, course, vacation, or other event, at times something seems to put a "spanner in the works." It could be unforeseen circumstances such as illness, miscommunication, or lack of finances.

In fact, life can be like an out-of-control roller coaster. While some people choose to ride it through and enjoy the thrill and accept the status quo, others are totally freaked out and want to jump off. Some just grin and bear it until the ride comes to an end.

The remedies are like a safety net, there to catch us when needed, and help us to deal with whatever life throws our way, from minor to major events or illness. Sometimes the sting can be severe – like a bungee chord unexpectedly snapping and slapping you hard in the face. One can either learn from that or just sit back and let it happen, or better prepared next time to do something about it and become a stronger person.

The following scenarios illustrate this. Two of them deal with coping with middle age, one with the reactions from being diagnosed with cancer, and the third one shows how differently people react to a particular event (each remedy personality type).

All in all the remedies are there for us when needed. In fact I was explaining to someone today what a week I have had. Two events did not go as planned—a lost or stolen item—the other, an event coming up in which I am preparing myself for the worst. Their answer – take some remedies!

Desperate Daunted Dada

The middle-aged man was celebrating his birthday. His present to himself was a fancy, shiny, fast sports car. Yes, the predictably red kind, he knew that, and yes it was bought to lessen the blow of his mid-life crisis.

Taking his new vehicle for a spin down the highway, he felt exhilarated. The open road in front—yup, this is the life, he thought. As the wind blew through his hair, in his reflection in the rear-view mirror, he noticed the widow peaks appearing. With a sigh, he thought, "Great! The hair jester has been poking fun at me."

Thinking back about the remarks from his young son – asking if his hair was falling out in clumps or just little by little – he began to feel a bit depressed. It was all right for his son. He had an exciting career mapped out for himself.

The thoughts of yesteryear returned; fun fishing trips with the boys, fancy motorboats, financial freedom to go where you pleased, and an exciting job. What now? What did he have to show for his life thus far?

Feeling even more depressed he decided to park the car and go for a walk to clear his head. It was a sunny day and he probably needed the exercise anyway. Yup, old age was certainly creeping in.

Walking down a windy road, he began to lose his way. There was no one to ask for directions so he carried on. Besides, even if there had been somebody to ask, he probably would not have asked. By the side of the road was a lone **Wild Oat** swaying in the wind, it was as though it was trying to point him in the right direction.

Suddenly things began to seem clearer, and he thought, "Why have I not thought of that before?" The skip had begun to return to his step, and the foggy future ahead began to lift.

The sun was beating down, so he sat under an **Oak** tree for a rest. Lying back admiring how the sturdy tree supported all the branches he started to drift off. He thought he heard someone whispering his name (or was he imagining it?) and telling him that instead of working so hard against all odds, he deserved to relax and have some fun.

Slowly, but surely, he got up and felt lighter. It was as if the weight of the world had been taken off his shoulders. Instead of purposeful strides, he was strolling at a relaxed pace, whistling a joyful tune, and admiring the wonders of nature.

A yellow flower (**Mimulus**) caught his eye and he bent down to take a closer look. He sniffed the flower and took a deep breath of relief. He had been feeling a bit tense and concerned of what old age would bring his way, but now he felt reassured that everything would work out fine.

Then something bizarre happened. He felt as if he had been hit on the head. He looked down and saw a **Walnut** that must just have blown off a tree. He examined it and again admired the cleverness of Mother Nature. The hard shell was protecting the soft nut inside. The old linked fence that was the divider between the future and his yesteryear was gradually melting away and he felt a free man. He would now be able to cope with the ageing process, and the snide comments from his son.

He had lost all track of time, and had without realizing it, walked in a circle. In the distance a crowd of people admired his new pride and joy. One of the older-looking men said, "That is a fine car you have there Sir. It is exactly what I have been looking for."

"Tell you what," he said. "Give me a ride home and a wad of cash and it is yours. I don't need it anymore". Grinning from ear to ear, and whistling quietly to himself all the way home, he felt a new man.

Mamma's Menopausal Madness

Do you want to feel like a spring chicken, and try to forget what your out-of-control body is doing to you? Want to look hot and not feel hot?

Forget about the madness that menopause brings. Exercise will bring a beautiful glow to your face. It will make a change from a hot powerful red face that your haywire body is subjecting you to. Red of all colours. How embarrassing! Why not a tan colour, a light coral pink? Why beetroot red?

Doesn't menopause mean a pause from men? So come and have a funky time with the girls. No need for makeup or a fancy hairdo. Forget about fashion and high-heeled shoes. Wear whatever feels comfortable. Anything loose fitting. An old pair of track pants, T-shirt, and trainers will do the trick.

Dance. Dance to the beat, joke around, and enjoy some time away from your everyday responsibilities. Remember the good old tunes from the swinging fifties and sixties. The Beatles and the Beach Boys. Have a giggle and a laugh. Life can be too serious sometimes. Laughter is the best medicine after all.

Dance to the right, dance to the left, and loosen up. Get caught up in the music, dream about being on a Yellow Submarine and immerse yourself into a time and place away from everything. The Beach Boys with take you to California, where you can soak up the warm yellow rays of sunshine. Tan yourself by the pool, swim in the crystal clear, topaz water.

Come back week after week to relax and rejuvenate in another time and place.

The Word "Cancer"

The word cancer creates a sense of dread and fear. It brings with it feelings of having no control over your body. It is up to the doctors to diagnose you and tell you your chances of survival. You are poked and prodded, while having to put your trust in others and hope everything will be all right.

How do you tell your loved ones the bad news? Once you have plucked up the courage, just thinking about it makes your heart sink. A deep sinking feeling, like the Titanic sinking to the bottom of the ocean, although everyone thought it was unsinkable. Then you ask yourself, why me? I eat sensibly, exercise regularly, and have never had any health problems in the past. Can my heart sink any deeper?

How will my loved ones take the news? Will they put on a brave face, or just crack and burst into tears? Will the tears be held back or will the floodgates open and keep pouring out like Niagara Falls?

Feelings of terror, unknown and known fears. What can help to alleviate my fears? Ah, the gentle Bach Flower Remedies that are made simply from flower petals floating on water, and energized by the sun. Ever so gently they work to help us regain a sense of courage and calmness and make us feel as if a huge weight has been lifted away.

The shock is like a strong electric current running through you. Ah yes, **Star of Bethlehem** can help, as it is the comforter and soother of pains and sorrows. This beautiful flower is like a star of hope way up in the sky. Don't forget to make a wish.

The thoughts just do not stop going around and around in my head, like an out-of-control record player. They are worrying thoughts that do not allow you to rest and go to sleep. Thank goodness, **White Chestnut** can assist with a peace of mind and a good night's rest.

Lastly, we must not forget about **Rescue Remedy**. This remedy is a truly a magical potion. Just take four drops and all the stress, fear, and worry melt away like snow in the sunshine. Thank you, Dr. Bach, for your wonderful remedies.

I know that the remedies cannot cure cancer, but they can help to put things into perspective and let your body heal itself the best it can.

The Special Meeting

It was a bigger crowd than they had expected, and it seemed as though lots of people had come "out of the woodwork" to see what all the fuss was about.

Vine was there surrounded by his "foot soldiers," for he was the one who had been wronged, and just needed to spread the word further to gain sympathy.

Cherry Plum arrived all nervous, heart beating, and ready to shout from the rooftops what had really happened.

Gentian was so discouraged and despondent, she sat with a glazed expression on her face.

Heather was just there for the company, and more concerned about talking to others about their latest ailment in graphic detail.

Holly, full of anger and hatred, was ready to pounce at any time.

Honeysuckle sat in a daze, thinking of the good old days and how things used to be.

Impatiens wanted things to get a move on, fidgeted and drummed his feet on the floor.

Mustard was so depressed he just sat there under his own cloud of misery.

Oak had been working in the background trying to make everyone get together and settle things "out of court" as it were.

Pine felt guilty and blamed himself.

Scleranthus could not decide which side they were on, nor where to sit, so stood at the back.

Star of Bethlehem was shocked and traumatized by the whole situation.

Water Violet came in and sat amongst her friends, heart beating. She sat silently holding onto her Bach Flower Kit.

Willow full of resentment, had compiled a long list of wrongdoings and sat near the back.

You could feel the tension, and the air could have been cut with a knife.

Vine and his buddies on one side, and the alleged wrongdoers and friends on the other.

Order was called by **Agrimony**, appearing jolly and cheerful, yet shaking inside.

The meeting did not go well. **Cerato** took over, but could not make up her mind who was in charge and how the meeting was to proceed.

Everyone had their say pointing their finger at the other. Voting here and voting there – nobody could decide what to do! Bedlam had arrived, and order had been lost.

Recess was called so everyone could take a deep breath, and gather their thoughts together. After the recess, everything seemed to have changed.

Vine stood up, and spoke on behalf of himself for a change. From now on, he boomed, let bygones be bygones and let us all work together as one.

Cerato called the meeting to order, and all was well.

Agrimony was happy and cracking jokes.

Cherry Plum was pleased that she had managed to control herself.

Gentian felt so much better and patted everyone on the back.

Heather was so stunned and happy at the outcome she was speechless.

Holly was being kind and sympathetic.

Honeysuckle went around taking photos of everyone.

Impatiens sat still and was overjoyed.

Mustard was overwrought with joy and happiness.

Oak went for a long-earned drink.

Pine felt great.

Scleranthus quickly decided to go for a drink with the others.

Star of Bethlehem was so relieved; they jumped up and down with joy.

Willow tore up his binder of all the evidence.

Water Violet went around calmly giving her blessings to all.

And finally...

So long my friend, it has been a pleasure sharing my insights and Bach Flower "reflections" with you.

And remember...

"Health depends on being in harmony with our souls"
(Dr. Edward Bach 1932)

Bibliography

The Twelve Healers and Other Remedies by Edward Bach, M.B., B.S., M.R.C.S., L.R.C.P., D.P.H.
First published in 1933 by The C.W. Daniel Company Ltd, England

The Bach Flower Remedies – Illustrations and Preparations by Nora Weeks and Victor Bullen
First published in 1964 by The C.W. Daniel Company Ltd, England

The 38 Flower Remedies – An Introduction and Guide to the 38 Flower Remedies
First published in 1995 by Wigmore Publications Ltd, England

Questions & Answers – The Bach Flower Remedies by John Ramsell
First published in 1986 by The C.W. Daniel Company Ltd, England

Further Information

For more information about the remedies, to order this book, or to sign up for a free monthly newsletter go to:
www.bachflowerscanada.com
info@bachflowerscanada.com

For further information about the remedies, advice, training courses, and more contact:
The Dr. Edward Bach Centre
Mount Vernon
Baker's Lane
Brightwell-cum-Sotwell
Oxon, OX10 0PZ, UK
00 44 (0)1491 834678
www.bachcentre.com

About the Author

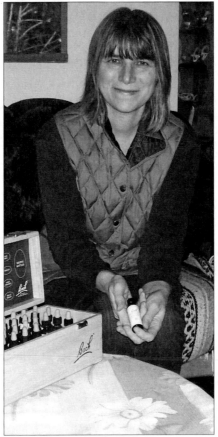

Photo taken by Josie Brune

Sarah Brune is a Bach Foundation Registered Practitioner (BFRP) and runs a successful Bach Flower business, **Inner Harmony Healing**, in the Comox Valley, BC, Canada. She has been using and working with the Bach Flower Remedies for many years. She lives in the Comox Valley, with her husband, two children, and two dogs.

Bach Foundation
REGISTERED PRACTITIONER

Index

A

Agrimony, 24,31,35,67,68
Animals, 9,11,12
Aspen, 31,36

B

Beech, 28,29,30,31,36

C

Case histories, 19
Centaury, 22,31,37
Cerato, 31,38,67,68
Cherry Plum, 9,20,31,39,66,68
Chestnut Bud, 12,18,22,25,28,
29,31,39
Chicory, 28,31,40
Clematis, 9,31,41
Consultations, 15,19,21,22
Crab Apple, 10,27,32,41

D

Dr. Edward Bach, 3,5,6,70

E

Elm, 20,22,23,25,29,32,42

G

Gentian, 24,32,43,66,68
Gorse, 32,43

H

Heather, 25,26,32,44,66,68
Holly, 12,28,29,30,32,45,66,68
Honeysuckle, 29,32,46,66,68
Hornbeam, 20,23,25,32,46,47

I

Impatiens, 9,25,28,32,47,66,68

L

Larch, 20,22,24,32,48

M

Mimulus, 12,18,22,24,32,48,63
Mustard, 29,30,33,49,66,68

O

Oak, 22,23,50,67,68
Olive, 20,25,28,33,50

P

Pine, 28,33,51,67,68,

R

Red Chestnut, 4,33,52
Reference chart, 31
Rescue Cream, 11,12

Rescue Remedy, 9,11,12,13,23,66
Rock Rose, 9,20,29,33,52
Rock Water, 33,53,

S

Scleranthus, 23,24,33,54,67,68
Star of Bethlehem, 9,29,33,55,
67,68
Sweet Chestnut, 20,24,33,55

V

Vervain, 12,18,25,33,56
Vine, 12,29,34,57,66,67

W

Walnut, 12,18,19,20,23,24,25,
28,29,30,34,57,64
Water Violet, 34,58,67,68
White Chestnut, 23,24,34,59,66
Wild Oat, 20,23,24,27,34,59,63
Wild Rose, 24,28,29,30,34,60
Willow, 20,22,24,29,34,60,61,
67,68